Hospital Transformation

Derek Burke • Prasad Godbole
Andrew Cash

Editors

Hospital Transformation

From Failure to Success and Beyond

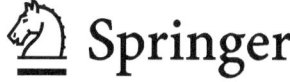

Editors
Derek Burke
Sheffield Children's NHS Foundation
Trust
Department of Emergency Medicine
Sheffield
UK

Prasad Godbole
Sheffield Children's NHS Foundation
Trust
Department of Paediatric Surgery
Sheffield
UK

Andrew Cash
Sheffield Teaching Hospitals NHS
Foundation Trust
Sheffield
UK

ISBN 978-3-030-15447-9   ISBN 978-3-030-15448-6   (eBook)
https://doi.org/10.1007/978-3-030-15448-6

This Springer imprint is published by the registered company Springer Nature Switzerland AG
The registered company address is: Gewerbestrasse 11, 6330 Cham, Switzerland

Foreword

This book is about balancing the sometimes-competing pressures of providing safe, high-quality hospital care within whatever resources a community is prepared to provide or the patient [or their insurer] is willing to pay. Throw into the mix the need for a learning culture, staff satisfaction, harmonious and effective team working, a good patient experience and high public esteem and the authors are searching for the illusive gold standard of hospital care and how to achieve it. Their search is internationally based and draws on research and evaluative studies from many countries.

Although the focus of the work is transforming hospitals, it gets deep into the wider policy and structural issues that frame the context in which hospitals have to perform. The contrast between a modern hospital in a developed society and one in a war-torn country is striking. Both are striving to achieve the best that is possible with the resources available to them.

The early chapters describe in some detail the various regulatory frameworks into which hospitals have to sit. Regulators play an increasingly important role, alongside health professional bodies, in setting standards which the successful hospital must attain. Some standards such as those relating to building and environmental safety are relatively clear but others such as adopting only evidence-based medicine across the whole organisation are more challenging, more fluid and sometimes more controversial. The best regulators and systems of accreditation are moving from inspection and compliance to systems of continuous improvement.

Different models of funding health systems are described and their strengths and weaknesses examined. Providing affordable health care to the poor and minority groups is a common challenge. Those countries such as Chile which have moved from one system to another provide a fascinating insight into the politics of health policy.

Although focused on success, the authors also examine why hospitals fail or find their standards dropping. How a hospital reacts to a change in economic circumstances without compromising its quality standards is an ever-present challenge for hospital managers and the leaders of health professions. In every country the gap between what medicine can achieve and what can be afforded appears to be growing. Hospitals and their specialist staff are usually at the leading edge of this challenge. Measuring clinical quality can be particularly demanding and the authors discuss means of identifying and dealing with unacceptable variations in clinical outcome.

Leadership is vital to sustained transformation. The most successful leaders build organisations that reflect a high degree of professional consensus about their aims and objectives. Their standards are often set higher than those specified by their external regulators. Strong leadership is diffused throughout the organisation, but the individuals concerned share the same attitudes and objectives. Medical leadership and particularly the role of the Medical Director is examined in some detail as is the concept of clinical governance. The best hospital organisations commonly have a high commitment to professional and nonprofessional training. This commitment usually means that the organisation is more open to regular internal challenge and new ideas.

Case studies drawn from both local and country-wide settings illuminate the text. An Australian case study examines the role of hospital boards. The UK study highlights the need for long-term but flexible plans to shape the future and provide the skilled human resources upon which success will be dependant.

Hospitals do not exist in a static world. In developed societies they have to adjust to increasingly elderly populations, constant and sometimes startling scientific change as well as economic and political pressures. The emergence of gene therapies and tailor-made medicines are but two examples. Every new scientific development usually leads to increased cost and new demand. Patient expectation almost always keeps pace with new science. Health professions will always want to deploy their new skills and patients want to benefit. It's almost a perfect storm!

Integrated health care is now widely accepted as the hallmark of excellent clinical practice. This means that the hospital and its staff have to find ways to blend their skills with others who are providing care and support including those in primary care and public health. This has to be done both at a community level and at the level of each patient. The authors drive home the point that biomedicine does not provide all the answers. Social care, family cohesion, housing, employment and poverty all impact on the health of communities. Hospitals need to play their part in the development of systems of health care as well as being centres for the treatment of illness.

The authors consider how successful hospitals begin the process of constant transformation. They distinguish between changes that produce short-term gain and those that imbed long-lasting quality changes into the core of the hospital. 'This is how we do it here is a powerful motto'. Successful hospitals almost always have patients at the core of both professional practice and managerial culture.

This book illustrates clearly how complex modern hospital organisations have become. But it also provides grounds to be confident that with the right leadership they can cope well with the tensions and challenges they face. It's not easy but it can be done.

Each chapter is well referenced for readers who want to explore beyond the words and ideas set out by the authors.

This work deserves a place on the book shelf of everybody involved in the hospital world. It's a '*keep going back to*' book as health professionals, managers, politicians and patients continue the search for that illusive gold standard.

Brian Edwards
Former President of European Hospital Federation
Emeritus Professor of Health Care Development
University of Sheffield
Sheffield, UK

Delivering high-quality healthcare services is predicated on achieving a balance between the cost of providing the service, the income derived from delivering that service (productivity and performance) and maintaining quality and safety.

A 'successful' hospital is one which can achieve the care standards stipulated by their regulators and at the same time deliver a financially robust service with excellent outcomes and patient experience.

The increasing burden of chronic illness combined with increased life expectancy due to advances in medicine and innovative technologies is putting a financial strain on many healthcare organisations. Patient awareness and expectations of better outcomes and experience is rising at the same time as the political imperative is to constrain costs. This conflict can tend to sway the balance towards services that become more focussed on balancing the books rather than on patient safety and quality. It is in such circumstances that hospitals may find themselves in a downward spiral of increasing costs and/or deterioration in the level of safety and performance with management conflicted as to how to turn this situation around.

This book addresses these issues with a global perspective. Individual chapters along with case studies where applicable give an insight into the challenge that healthcare organisations face on a global scale. The transformation and turnaround process and sustainability following transformation with practical examples are also addressed. All chapters can be read as standalone or sequentially.

The book is aimed at all healthcare staff, particularly those in leadership positions and in managerial roles whether clinical or non-clinical.

We would like to take the opportunity to thank our esteemed team of contributors for their timely submission of their contributions without which this book would have been impossible. We are grateful for the support and guidance of Melissa Morton, Executive Editor at Springer Science and Business Media, and Prakash Marudhu Project Coordinator for Springer Nature.

Finally, we would like to thank our families who have supported and encouraged us through this venture without which this would not have been possible.

Sheffield, UK	Derek Burke
Sheffield, UK	Prasad Godbole
Sheffield, UK	Andrew Cash

Contents

Contributors

Derek Burke Department of Emergency Medicine, Sheffield Children's NHS Foundation Trust, Sheffield, UK

Andrew Cash Sheffield Teaching Hospitals NHS Foundation Trust, Sheffield, UK

Patrick Dobbs Sheffield Teaching Hospitals NHS Foundation Trust, Sheffield, UK

Stephen Duckett Grattan Institute, Carlton, VIC, Australia

Prasad Godbole Department of Paediatric Surgery, Sheffield Children's NHS Foundation Trust, Sheffield, UK

Christine Jorm NSW Regional Health Partners, Newcastle, NSW, Australia

Martin A. Koyle The Hospital for Sick Children (SickKids), Toronto, ON, Canada

Department of Surgery, University of Toronto School of Medicine, Toronto, ON, Canada

Matthew Kurian Doncaster and Bassetlaw NHS Foundation Trust, Doncaster, UK

Dawn Lawson Liverpool Health Partners, Liverpool, UK

Jaime Llambías-Wolff York University, Toronto, ON, Canada

Erwin Loh Monash Centre for Health Research and Implementation, Monash University, Clayton, VIC, Australia

Katherine Lorenz Monash Centre for Health Research and Implementation, Monash University, Clayton, VIC, Australia

Stephen Stericker Care to Innovate, NHS and Social Care, York, UK

Rivanna Stuhler The Hospital for Sick Children (SickKids), Toronto, ON, Canada

The Institute for Health Policy, Management, and Evaluation (IHPME), University of Toronto, Toronto, ON, Canada

Tim Tomlinson Pioneer Healthcare Limited, Sheffield, UK

Part I

Requirements of Basic Healthcare Globally

Prasad Godbole

Introduction

Every individual has a right to basic healthcare. With increasing patient awareness and expectation, it goes without saying that hospitals have to deliver healthcare that is patient focused, meets the demands of the patients, is provided in collaboration with patient views and is cost effective. Anyone going into hospital does so with the inherent notion of receiving safe treatment. However how can patient safety be guaranteed? It is here that hospitals have to adhere to regulatory requirements. Regulations are there irrespective of the model of healthcare delivery:

A. To ensure that the hospitals themselves provide a safe environment in which to work and provide treatment—structural regulations, licensing and accreditation
B. The systems and processes in hospitals are such that patients will receive safe treatment—licensing and accreditation
C. To ensure that Doctors and nurses treating the patients have the appropriate qualifications and experience—medical regulatory authorities
D. To ensure that the best evidence is used when treating patients—compliance with National Guidelines or international guidelines

E. To ensure quality assurance and patient focused healthcare delivery as well as financial integrity

Where any of these regulatory processes are not complied with, inevitably patient safety will be compromised.

Is Regulation of Healthcare Services Truly Global?

In both the developed and developing countries, there is regulation of healthcare service provision. While this regulation exists, the implementation and adherence to regulation may vary depending on the geopolitical climate. For example in war torn countries, regulation although present cannot necessarily be monitored when the prime task of the workforce is to save lives in the most inhospitable conditions. Furthermore in certain developing countries where it is difficult to access any sort of healthcare, alternative medical practitioners may practice traditional allopathic medicine with scant regard to the regulations. Even in developed countries such as the U.K. male non therapeutic circumcisions are undertaken in the community by general practitioners and religious leaders with very little audit or control of outcomes or facilities where they are undertaken (https://www.bma.org.uk/advice/employment/ethics/children-and-young-people/male-circumcision). In Africa although

P. Godbole (✉)
Department of Paediatric Surgery, Sheffield Children's NHS Foundation Trust, Sheffield, UK
e-mail: Prasad.Godbole@sch.nhs.uk

© Springer Nature Switzerland AG 2019
D. Burke et al. (eds.), *Hospital Transformation*, https://doi.org/10.1007/978-3-030-15448-6_1

female genital mutilation is illegal, this is still practiced on cultural grounds (http://www.who.int/news-room/fact-sheets/detail/female-genital-mutilation). This highlights the fact that while regulations for hospitals may be global, the implementation and monitoring to achieve global patient safety is far from ideal.

Structural Regulations

For any new healthcare facility, each country has a specific building code for civil works. For hospital design, functional space planning guidelines are available which outline interdependencies, co adjacencies and functional flow. Regulations for fire safety, HVAC (heating, ventilation and air conditioning), electromechanical configurations exist. These regulatory codes are most commonly used for new hospital builds and can be used for the commissioning process of new builds. These codes also include room data sets with finishing and fittings. Examples of this are the Health Building Notes (HBN) (https://assets.publishing.service.gov.uk/government/uploads/system/uploads/attachment_data/file/316247/HBN_00-01-2.pdf), ASHE guidelines (http://www.ashe.org), International Health Planning Guidance (https://www.wbdg.org/building-types/health-care-facilities/hospital) and local civil and building regulations for hospitals such as the Indian Code for Hospital Builds (https://archive.org/details/gov.in.is.12433.1.1988/page/n5).

Licensing and Accreditation

Accreditation is usually a voluntary program, sponsored by a non-governmental organization (NGO), in which trained external peer reviewers evaluate a healthcare organization's compliance and compare it with pre-established performance standards [1]. Quality standards for hospitals and other medical facilities were first introduced in the United States in the "Minimum Standard for Hospitals" developed by the American College of Surgeons in 1917. After World War

II, increased world trade in manufactured goods led to the creation of the International Standards Organization (ISO) in 1947 [2]. Accreditation formally started in the United States with the formation of the Joint Commission on Accreditation of Healthcare Organizations (JCAHO) in 1951. This model was exported to Canada and Australia in the 1960s and 1970s and reached Europe in the 1980s. Accreditation programs spread all over the world in the 1990s [3]. There are other forms of systems used worldwide to regulate, improve and market the services of healthcare providers and organizations, including Certification and Licensure. Certification involves formal recognition of compliance with set standards (e.g., ISO 9000 standards) validated by external evaluation by an authorized auditor. Licensure involves a process by which governmental authority grants permission, usually following inspection against minimal standards, to an individual practitioner or healthcare organization to operate in an occupation or profession [3]. Although the terms accreditation and certification are often used interchangeably, accreditation usually applies only to organizations, while certification may apply to individuals, as well as to organizations [2]. In summary, licensing is a mandatory regulatory requirement for hospitals and individuals to practise. Accreditation has been shown to improve the quality of healthcare outcomes [4] and is voluntary e.g. Joint Committee International (JCI) (https://www.jointcommissioninternational.org) accreditation of hospitals or departments.

Medical Regulatory Authorities

For any doctor or nurse to practice, they have to have gained the appropriate qualification and experience and been registered with their country's medical or nursing medical authority. This registration may or may not be transferable from one country to the other. For example the basic medical qualification from India is not recognised in the European Countries or the US and doctors have to complete that country's qualifying exams to enable them to get further training and license/certificate to practice once the performance standards are achieved. In certain countries like the U.K. doctors have to undergo a process of revalidation every 5 years (https://www.england.nhs.uk/medical-revalidation/doctors/10-steps/) to ensure that they remain up to date with no concerns to the public about their competence or performance. Similarly doctors and nurses from non English speaking countries (excluding EU countries) have to pass an English proficiency test prior to working in the U.K. (https://www.ielts.org).

Evidence Based Medicine and Regulation

It is estimated that upto 48 million Americans suffer from chronic pain daily leading to an estimated cost per annum of between $560 and 635 million [5] and loss of productivity [6]. It was long thought that opioids prescribed for chronic pain did not cause addiction, however this has now shown to be untrue [7]. The CDC issued guidance on prescribing opioids for chronic pain [8]. Similarity the National Institute for Health and Care Excellence (NICE) (https://www.nice.org.uk) publishes evidence based guidance for which there is a mandatory reporting requirement for hospitals to demonstrate compliance.

Quality Assurance and Regulation

The regulatory requirements regarding quality assurance vary from country to country. While many countries have a mandatory requirement to publish outcomes for key conditions such as cancer treatment, joint replacements etc., many countries do not publish such data. Furthermore in countries where many clinicians are private practitioners, there may not be auditable data of their practice despite regulations being in place. In certain regions of the world, quality assurance is non existent. From personal experience, this situation is prevalent in war torn countries.

In the U.K. every NHS Trust is mandated to provide a safety thermometer (https://www.safetythermometer.nhs.uk) or dashboard as well as outcomes by individual hospital and clinician. Key reporting requirements include incidence of MRSA, C. Difficile, hospital acquired urinary tract infections, deep vein thrombosis, pressure ulcers etc.

Furthermore every hospital in the U.K. that have been given Foundation Trust status (status to operate independent of government control) is licensed by Monitor (https://www.gov.uk/government/organisations/monitor) and regulated by the Care Quality Commission (https://www.cqc.org.uk). The focus of the CQC is primarily patient safety, patient focus and experience and quality and effectiveness. Hospitals are rated from outstanding to inadequate and where appropriate hospitals may be put into special measures to enable a hospital turnaround process to be undertaken. These regulatory mechanisms also oversee financial integrity of the institutions who are given a financial risk rating [9].

Conclusion

There are certain key regulatory requirements for any healthcare provider globally. These include regulatory frameworks from hospital build to patient care and regulations for all individuals providing the care. However these regulatory frameworks are not consistent or standardised and it is therefore imperative that there is collaboration on a global scale to ensure patient safety.

References

1. Shaw CD. Toolkit for accreditation programs. The International Society for Quality in Health Care, Australia; 2004.
2. Montagu D. Accreditation and other external quality assessment systems for healthcare: review of experience and lessons learned. London: Department for International Development Health Systems Resource Centre. Available from: http://www.dfidhealthrc.org/publications/health_service_delivery/Accreditation.pdf. Accessed 2003.
3. Shaw CD. External quality mechanisms for health care: summary of the ExPeRT project on visitatie, accreditation, EFQM and ISO assessment in European Union countries. External peer review techniques. European foundation for quality management.

International organization for standardization. Int J Qual Health Care. 2000;12:169–75.

4. Alkhenizan A, Shaw C. Impact of accreditation on the quality of healthcare services: a systematic review of the literature. Ann Saudi Med. 2011;31(4):407–16.

5. Nahin Richard L. Estimates of pain prevalence and severity in adults: United States, 2012. J Pain. 2015;16(8):769–80.

6. Institute of Medicine (US) Committee on Advancing Pain Research, Care, and Education. Relieving pain in America: a blueprint for transforming prevention, care, education, and research. Washington, DC: National Academies Press; 2011.

7. Banta-Green CJ, Merrill JO, Doyle SR, Boudreau DM, Calsyn DA. Opioid use behaviors, mental health and pain-development of a typology of chronic pain patients. Drug Alcohol Depend. 2009;104:34–42.

8. Dowell D, Haegerich T, Chou R, et al. CDC guideline for prescribing opioids for chronic pain. United States, 2016. MMWR Recomm Rep. 2016;65(1):1–49.

9. The regulation and oversight of NHS trusts and NHS foundation trusts. Joint policy statement to accompany care bill quality of services clauses. Available at https://assets.publishing.service.gov.uk/government/uploads/system/uploads/attachment_data/file/200446/regulation-oversight-NHS-trusts.pdf.

Tim Tomlinson and Prasad Godbole

Introduction

The world continues to become a smaller place made possible by growing access to Internet, online services and less expensive air travel. An increasing number of developing countries are experiencing economic growth far in excess of previous years with real growth in GDP at rate well above the levels in the recognised developed world of USA and Europe [1]. The period of austerity continues its grip and the gap between the Middle East previously seen as cash rich is narrowing as the reliance on oil as the main source of energy reduces. There are now wide opportunities across the globe to partner with governments and private providers aspiring to develop healthcare to levels of international standards. However, the challenges of global healthcare remain significant. Dr. Margaret Chan, Director General of the WHO states:

> We want to see better health and well-being for all, as an equal human right. Money does not buy better health. Good policies that promote equity have a better chance. We must tackle the root causes (of ill health and inequities) through a social determinants approach that engages the whole of government and the whole of society.

T. Tomlinson
Pioneer Healthcare Limited, Sheffield, UK
e-mail: ttomlinson@pioneerhealthcare.co.uk

P. Godbole (✉)
Department of Paediatric Surgery, Sheffield
Children's NHS Foundation Trust, Sheffield, UK
e-mail: Prasad.Godbole@sch.nhs.uk

All individuals equate high quality healthcare with a good quality of life. This is at the forefront of most governments thinking and ranks highest alongside the economy as a political issue. In the U.K., the National Health Service has faced significant challenges in continuing to provide healthcare free at the point of delivery.

This chapter will discuss the challenges facing global healthcare and the opportunities that have arisen as a result with the aim of providing a consistent, high quality healthcare to basic minimum standards. The chapter is based on literature but also personal experience of the authors in the delivery of international healthcare.

Global Healthcare Challenges

Population Demographics and Disease Pattern

It is well known that people are living longer thanks to emerging new technologies and advances in science. The average life expectancy of the population in the OECD countries is approximately 80 years (https://www.oecd.org/berlin/47570143.pdf). However in many cases, this increased life expectancy is linked to chronic disease requiring lifelong treatment [2].

Globally, the rate of deaths from noncommunicable causes, such as heart disease, stroke, and injuries, is growing. At the same time, the number of deaths from infectious diseases, such as

© Springer Nature Switzerland AG 2019
D. Burke et al. (eds.), *Hospital Transformation*, https://doi.org/10.1007/978-3-030-15448-6_2

malaria, tuberculosis, and vaccine-preventable diseases, is decreasing [3]. Many developing countries must now deal with a "dual burden" of disease [4]: they must continue to prevent and control infectious diseases, while also addressing the health threats from noncommunicable diseases and environmental health risks. As social and economic conditions in developing countries change and their health systems and surveillance improve, more focus will be needed to address noncommunicable diseases, mental health, substance abuse, eating disorders and especially, injuries (both intentional and unintentional). Some countries are beginning to establish programs to address these issues. For example, Kenya has implemented programs for road traffic safety and violence prevention (http://www.who.int/violence_injury_prevention/road_traffic/countrywork/ken/en/).

Other countries are facing new issues. In China for example 400,000 new HIV cases have been seen in the last 12 months (WHO) [5]. Transmission of HIV was previously almost entirely caused by infected blood products which has been replaced by infection via sexual contact due in the main to legalisation of single sex relationships. With an associated cultural stigma of same sex relationships existing in China and noting that most men actually marry in to a heterosexual relationship the disease is affecting the male and female population.

While health promotion and developing healthy lifestyles is likely to have an impact on chronic disease in the long term, health economies will still face the burden of management and treatment for the affected generation. Obesity for example is becoming a major problem globally with its attended consequences including diabetes, cardiovascular and respiratory diseases.

A key challenge in many underdeveloped countries is to introduce primary care services as both provider and gatekeeper backed up by information/data to support a cost effective secondary and tertiary care system.

Expanding international trade introduces new health risks. A complex international distribution chain has resulted in potential international outbreaks due to food borne infections, poor quality pharmaceuticals, and contaminated consumer goods.

The world community is finding better ways to confront major health threats. WHO, through the 2005 IHR External Web Site Policy (http://www.who.int/ihr/procedures/implementation/en/), proposes new guidance and promotes cooperation between developed and developing countries on emerging health issues of global importance. The IHR require countries to develop appropriate surveillance and response capacities to address these health concerns. All of these issues will require internationally enhanced collaboration with other countries to protect and promote better health for all.

Cost Control

Promoting health in current times of austerity can be a daunting task. With more and more technologies emerging and the focus shifting to patient centred care and patient autonomy, it can be difficult to provide these technologies (sometimes experimental) to patients who demand it. Spending on healthcare outstrips the GDP of most countries in the developed world [6]. This combined with austerity measures and 'doing more for less' is a significant challenge facing most governments. With the complex interrelationships between insurers, hospitals and patients in countries where healthcare is not free, this can lead to differences in coverage of the population to various interventions. In some of the GCC countries, this has led to marked differences in what healthcare interventions will be paid for by the insurers and what the patients themselves have to pay for.

Human Resources and the Workforce

Staff in most of Haiti's 19 public hospitals have been on strike for a long time (https://www.dailymail.co.uk/wires/ap/article-4137896/Staff-strikes-shutter-Haitis-public-hospitals.html), Jamaica is in the midst of a health care crisis as specialised nurses leave the country en masse for jobs in North America and Europe (http://www. loopjamaica.com/content/nurses-exodus-continues-uk-now-big-drawing-card) and in Kenya, a massive strike among doctors demanding better working conditions has left millions of people without access to any government provided health care (https://www.bbc.co.uk/news/world-africa-39271850) and this situation has only recently been resolved.

The global shortage of health workers is getting worse [7]. In many countries, doctors, nurses, midwives and others are left to burn out in bad working conditions—or leave their countries altogether—countries and their communities suffer then from loss of front line staff creating a negative spiral into lower-quality care.

Organisations are working to change this, but it will take time, investment, different ways of thinking and a new generation of aid.

Proper management of human resources is critical in providing a high quality of health care. A refocus on human resources management in health care and more research is needed to develop new policies. Effective human resources management strategies are greatly needed to achieve better outcomes from and access to health care around the world.

Internationally the recruitment and retention of healthcare professionals is becoming more difficult year on year as demand continues to outstrip supply in competition with what are seen as more lucrative less pressured forms of employment in areas such as IT.

In the U.K. the Brexit conundrum has left many of the European workforce uncertain of their longer term futures within the U.K. thereby exacerbating the existing shortages in nursing and medical workforce within the NHS.

Medical Education

The number of overseas students accessing university placements in U.K. gives opportunity to provide U.K. standard education in countries of origin. Establishing the delivery of training standards equivalent to but outside of U.K. is a challenge which requires joint initiatives probably at a government to government level. However, while training can be provided to a certain standard, implementation of those standards may not be possible in their country of origin either due to political uncertainty, geopolitical, cultural influences or financial uncertainty. This is more significant in countries that have been involved in war for many years. The author's visits to such countries have demonstrated a high level of skill of the workforce comparable to internationally acceptable standards but an impossible task of implementation of those standards as a result of in some cases a complete breakdown of structured society creating a total lack of clinical and administrative/operational level organisation. The current conflict in Syria is a prime example of this as skilled surgeons function in make shift accomodation [8].

Accessibility and Rationalisation of Healthcare Services

On a global scale, hospitals vary in size from polyclinics providing basic levels of care to large multi specialty hospitals. Continuing on from the theme of patient demand and supply as well as the increasing costs of running a hospital, closing smaller units or departments within units (more so within government sponsored organisations like the NHS) has been considered causing much public outcry. Centralisation of very specialised services is also an increasing feature of the rationalisation of services to maximise expertise and reduce the financial burden.

Quality and Outcome Measures

The focus of any healthcare system is on the quality of the service provided and the outcome measures of the interventions. This unfortunately is lacking in many developed countries where healthcare outcomes lag behind developed countries [9]. In the U.K. the National Health Service has developed a 'safety thermometer' which has to be reported on a monthly basis. Pressures sores, incidence of MRSA or other hospital acquired infections, C. Difficile, Deep vein thrombosis are a few of the general outcomes that have to be reported (https://www.safetythermom-eter.nhs.uk). Furthermore there has become a trend towards outcome reporting for certain key specialties which are available by individual specialist in the public domain. This is not the case globally. There are very few standard outcome measures reported on a consistent basis to allow for comparison or quality assurance of the health systems on an international platform. With the advent of the U.K. National Institute for Health and Clinical Effectiveness (NICE) (https://www.nice.org.uk) emphasis is being increased on clinical interventions which are effective and provide value for money. Increasingly commissioners of healthcare are using the guidelines published by NICE to effectively ration intereventions. This has been the case in terms of the surgical treatment of varicose veins some 10 years ago. However, a gradual increase in the number of varicose ulcers requiring long term often costly treatment is leading to a rethink in this strategy.

Patient Centric Healthcare

There is no doubt that all healthcare providers would agree that it is not only the outcomes that matter to the patients but also the overall patient experience [10]. Increasing awareness and knowledge amongst patients and their expectations should be catered to as 'customers' of the hospital. This awareness is increasing with increased reliance on social media. Feedback from patients is important and constructive criticism is desirable. A willingness of healthcare providers to act on this feedback is essential to maintain the quality of the service. Feedback from the workforce providing the service is also essential. A demoralised workforce will not necessarily provide the best quality of treatment. In the National Health Service, the Friends and Family Test (FFT) (https://www.england.nhs.uk/fft/) has been introduced as a comparator amongst NHS organisations. Where hospitals have failed, a root cause analysis has demonstrated a chronic failure by senior management to act on patient feedback or feedback from the hospital staff [11].

While the challenges are daunting, health challenges require active involvement of all levels of government (international, national, and local). In an interdependent world, the need to act together on health challenges and on the determinants of health becomes ever more important.

A partnership-based vision is required engaging with governments, nongovernmental organisations, civil society, the private sector, science and academics, health professionals, communities—and every individual citizen. How strongly leadership of this process emerges holds the key to future step changes.

Global Healthcare Opportunities

Investment

There is an increasing trend where countries with high economic growth enlist the assistance of reputed internationally recognised organisations to provide and improve the quality of healthcare in their region. The investment in this infrastructure may be by the government themselves or by non governmental organisations (NGO) [12]. The GCC countries is an example of this investment. The United Arab Emirates has seen an explosion of healthcare facilities with international collaboration.

The National Health Service has recognised this opportunity of exporting it's brand with the aim of improving the quality of healthcare internationally. Individual NHS Trusts may aim to do so as part of their strategic vision for international growth and a new revenue stream. Independent organisations may provide quality assurance systems as part of turnkey solutions to new hospital development projects with the aim of 'getting it right the first time'. The authors have experience of the latter in the GCC countries, Sub Saharan Africa and Far East Asia where there is an appetite and drive for healthcare improvement. The Moorfields eye hospital, an NHS Trust in London U.K. established a satellite hospital in Dubai in 2007, permanently staffed and providing outpatients and day care services for patients with eye conditions. The staff provide a high quality care at par with their U.K. parent hospital standards. They have undertaken over 30,000 patient episodes from the UAE and wider Middle East and are also active in research and education. In the U.K. organisations like UKIHMA (U.K. International Healthcare Management Association) (http://www.ukihma.co.uk) provides links between U.K. organisations and overseas clients. The UK Export Finance department (within the U.K. Treasury department) facilitates government to government loans or supports organisations with capital funding to provide healthcare services internationally. This trend is set to continue for the foreseeable future with the most recent budget (October 2018) providing an additional £2 billion towards UKEF funding going forward [13].

Teaching and Training

With the provision of international healthcare services, there is a significant element of teaching and training. This is not only in the sphere of clinical practice but also operational management of hospitals and in some instances commences from the concept and design phase of a new hospital project through to operational management. Clinical teaching and training is well established with specialists in their field being sought after to visit established institutions abroad to develop the skills framework for that institution specifically but the region at large. In the author's experience, this teaching and training has been very well received and disseminated to the workforce to ensure sustainability of the teaching program.

Research

There are three global priorities in global research. The first priority is to undertake research and service delivery of key basic healthcare needs namely clean water, sanitation, food, mosquito nets, maternal and child welfare, vaccines to name a few. The second priority is to develop research strategies to tackle the growing problems with smoking, obesity, diabetes and cardiovascular disease. The final priority is development of new technologies and treatments. International collaboration in research studies and multi institutional clinical trials are a significant opportunity for independent researchers and research institutes to promote health and well being globally [14].

Careers

Organisational opportunities in international markets has already been referred to above. Hand in hand with this is the opportunity to develop and enhance one's career. It is well known that markets such as the Philippines and India 'export' high quality nurses overseas, especially in the Middle East giving them the financial stability and career trajectory that may not be available in their own country. Similarly opportunities for clinicians and allied healthcare workers are significant in the healthcare market. With ease of travel making no destination in the world out of bounds, more and more doctors are able to undertake further training overseas or provide their expertise in markets where this is required. This also brings the opportunity to have a career, certainly as a Physician or surgeon which spans more than one country or continent.

Conclusion

International healthcare provision remains a challenge in terms of accessibility, finance, cost effectiveness, patient demand and consistency of outcomes. There remains significant variability in the delivery of patient care to a basic minimum standard and quality. Healthcare needs to be more patient centred, evidence based and transparent. Numerous opportunities exist to achieve these deliverables; however, these require close government to government relationships and a willingness to put healthcare at the forefront of key priorities.

References

1. World economic situation and prospects 2018. United Nations. Available at https://www.un.org/development/desa/dpad/wp-content/uploads/sites/45/publication/WESP2018_Full_Web-1.pdf.
2. Crimmins EM. Lifespan and healthspan: past, present, and promise. Gerontologist. 2015;55(6):901–11.
3. Ediriweerar DS, Karunapema P, Pathmeswaran A, Arnold M. Increase in premature mortality due to non-communicable diseases in Sri Lanka during the first decade of the twenty-first century. BMC Public Health. 2018;18:584.
4. Boutayeb A. The double burden of communicable and non-communicable diseases in developing countries. Trans R Soc Trop Med Hyg. 2006;100(3):191–9.
5. Choi KH, Liu H, Guo Y, Han L, Mandel JS, Rutherford GW. Emerging HIV-1 epidemic in China in men who have sex with men. Lancet. 2003;361(9375):2125–6.
6. Health spending in most OECD countries rises, with the U.S. far outstripping all others. Report of the OECD. Available at http://www.oecd.org/general/healthspendinginmostoecdcountriesriseswiththeusfaroutstrippingallothers.htm.
7. Darzi A, Evans T. The global shortage of health workers—an opportunity to transform care. Lancet. 2016;388(10060):2576–7.
8. Kherallah M, Alahfez T, Sahloul Z, Eddin KD, Jamil G. Health care in Syria before and during the crisis. Avicenna J Med. 2012;2(3):51–3.
9. Ruger JP, Kim HJ. Global health inequalities: an international comparison. J Epidemiol Community Health. 2006;60(11):928–36.
10. Yeoman G, Furlong P, Seres M, et al. Defining patient centricity with patients for patients and caregivers: a collaborative endeavour. BMJ Innov. 2017;3:76–83.
11. Report of the Mid Staffordshire NHS Foundation Trust Public Inquiry. Available at https://www.gov.uk/government/publications/report-of-the-mid-staffordshire-nhs-foundation-trust-public-inquiry.
12. Krech R, Kickbusch I, Franz C, et al. Banking for health: the role of financial sector actors in investing in global health. BMJ Glob Health. 2018;3:e000597.
13. Budget 2018: Philip Hammond's speech. Available at https://www.gov.uk/government/speeches/budget-2018-philip-hammonds-speech.
14. Research and innovation for global health transformation. Available at https://www.nihr.ac.uk/funding-and-support/global-health-research/funding-calls/research-and-innovation-for-global-health-transformation.htm.

Models of Healthcare in Developed and Developing Countries

Prasad Godbole and Matthew Kurian

Introduction

There are about 200 countries in the world all of whom deliver healthcare to their population. Although there are 200 countries, the models of healthcare delivery can broadly be classified into four basic models.

The Beveridge Model

The report by William Beveridge during the time of the Second World War (The Beveridge Report) (https://www.parliament.uk/about/living-heritage/transformingsociety/livinglearning/coll-9-health1/coll-9-health/) advocated a proactive approach by the public sector in promoting health of the people. The report became the foundation for the creation of the National Health Service (NHS), amongst the first health care system, free at the point of delivery and funded by tax. In this system, the healthcare is funded from general taxation, like any other public service like the police force or community libraries. Most hospitals are government owned, and most healthcare

P. Godbole (✉)
Department of Paediatric Surgery, Sheffield
Children's NHS Foundation Trust, Sheffield, UK
e-mail: Prasad.Godbole@sch.nhs.uk

M. Kurian
Doncaster and Bassetlaw NHS Foundation Trust,
Doncaster, UK

workers are employed by the government. Salaries are fixed and costs of treatments are standardised. In private hospitals that provide a service free at the point of delivery, the hospitals get paid by the government. As the government is the sole payor of all costs of healthcare treatment, it can control what the doctor can do and what the hospital can charge. This 'general taxation' model or a variation of this model is favoured in Great Britain, Scandinavian countries, New Zealand and Spain [1].

It is thought that having a central single system of general taxation 'under one roof' would bring efficiencies to the healthcare delivery due to economies of scale. However while this may be possible in theory due to less bureaucracy and administrative burden [2], in practice it is far from true. As part of the government, any administrative shortfalls within the government is likely to be to some degree replicated within the healthcare sector [3].

Furthermore financing of the healthcare service through general taxation can be challenging. With an ever increasing age of the population and increase in chronic diseases, more money needs to be found to fund this. Raising taxes is never a popular option with governments who therefore have to somehow economise in their service delivery.

In the NHS, the National Institute of Health and Care Excellence (NICE) (https://www.nice.org.uk/), provides guidance on best practices against which hospitals are scrutinised for compliance. Furthermore NICE can play the role of gatekeeper in determining which treatments are cost effective and should be provided.

While the patient never receives a bill, rationing to some extent of healthcare services may preclude some patients from receiving 'non urgent or non essential treatment'. Decentralisation and devolving of the budgets and decision making to local authorities and municipalities and councils may increase this rationing and may encourage those who can afford it to pay out of pocket for their treatment. In the U.K. Clinical Commissioning Groups led by primary care practitioners, non clinical managers and senior nurses are a prime example of this. It has become apparent these groups are many a times conflicted between cost saving, personal views and implementing what is seen as the best for the population. As a result certain groups have no service, and others have a greater focus. Conditions such as varicose veins, simple uncomplicated hernia repairs are not routinely funded unless by exception. This has gradually increased during the last decade and the prolonged period of austerity, a far cry from the previous decade when the Labour government opened the taps on spending in the NHS.

Earmarking specific areas of general taxation has been used to fund the general taxation model. For example in Australia the tax on tobacco is ploughed back into the healthcare system (https://www.dailymail.co.uk/news/article-5712033/How-smokers-paying-nations-health-care-17billion-paid-tobacco-taxes.html) and has been for a number of years. A similar earmarking arrangement is also in place in countries like Portugal, Finland and South Korea. In Brazil, the Unified Health System established in 1988 brought a huge population without healthcare into the fold. However chronic underfunding, lack of adequate workforce and equipment shortages have led to lengthy waits and for those with money to opt for private insurance based healthcare [4].

The Bismarck Model

Most notably found in Germany [5] this model is funded by an insurance system. Financing is provided by employers and employees through payroll deductions and covers the entire population. In Germany there are approximately 240 insurers, however contrary to the USA, these are not for profit. Due to the tight regulatory control by the Government, there is much better control over costs. In most cases, at least a significant proportion of the costs of the patient are reimbursed through these schemes. Most people will get additional private insurance to cover the top up reimbursement costs. While this is primarily aimed at employers and employees, those without jobs are supported by the government to get complete coverage.

However the risk of this model is the burden of tax on the employed population. In countries such as Belgium and France, the tax wedge on labor income is significant and can make the countries less competitive in the international market for attracting inbound employment [6].

The National Health Insurance Model

This system has elements of both the Beveridge and Bismarck Model. Every citizen pays into a government sponsored insurance program and healthcare is provided in the private sector [7]. Canada is a leading example of this system and the healthcare coverage is universal. As every citizen pays into the insurance program, there is no need for marketing or any incentives to deny any claims. Furthermore as a single payor, this can drive down costs through negotiations with vendors most notably in the pharmaceutical industry. While this system works, it may not cover every condition and there is a likelihood that patients may have to wait longer to be seen or to have treatment. Apart from Canada, Taiwan and South Korea are emerging markets that utilise this model [8].

Private Insurance and Out of Pocket Model

In many of the developing countries there is a vast gulf between the rich and the poor. In countries such as India, those with adequate finances can avail of the numerous private hospitals for their healthcare. In the 1980s there were only two options for healthcare in India. One was the government owned hospitals and the other was private healthcare for profit facilities. However over the last two decades there has been an insurgence of private insurance providing healthcare cover for those who can afford it [9]. However, those who are extremely poor or who have no or little access to healthcare have to somehow find the means to pay for their healthcare. Many of those who are unable to afford healthcare or do not have the means to access any healthcare either succumb to their illness or as in the past pay for healthcare by other means (paying in livestock is not unheard of even today). To maximise coverage of healthcare, the concept of corporate social responsibility is in place in India where big corporate organisations have by law to set aside a sum of money for infrastructure projects such as healthcare [10]. This health paradox in India is as diverse as the country and its different ethnic groups. It is served by traditional health resource, homeopathy and Ayurveda, and more conventional allopathic system. This is delivered by a poorly resourced and managed Government service, and a very advanced technology supported private health service. The private health service compares with the best in the world, and attracts health tourists from Europe and Africa. It even boasts of an organ transplant service sponsored by Corporate business houses. Population growth, and female literacy are the biggest challenges to delivery of health. The state of Kerala, that boasts 100% female literacy, has health parameters that can compare with the best in the world. Assistance of voluntary organisations, in health delivery, has helped eradicate polio from the country.

It has long been thought that by encouraging private insurance would lessen the burden of healthcare provision on governments. However most private insurers are for profit and hence can decide to refuse coverage for preexisting conditions or other conditions with a view to minimising claims and maximising profit. Furthermore, it is likely that doctors may over investigate or prescribe for insured patients on the assumption that the insurer will pay for it. Furthermore, those

with ill health and can afford to do so are likely to take out private insurance policies for their healthcare and more likely to claim for this thereby increasing the premium for healthy individuals with private insurance.

In the U.K. private health insurance may be self funded or through employers. Self pay packages for treatments are also available. However in some instances, private or self pay initial consultations may be requested with a view to bypassing the wait for an outpatient appointment and potentially (but not necessarily ethically) fast track their subsequent treatment in the public sector. Many developing countries have to some degree a combination of out of pocket and private insurance healthcare model. However the majority of the global population where healthcare infrastructure is scarce, the government in turmoil or in crisis, in war torn regions, the out of pocket model remains in place for millions of people.

What about the U.S.A.?

The United States is exemplified by a somewhat disjointed delivery of healthcare using all four models. The U.S.A. has the highest per capita expenditure on healthcare than any of the OECD countries [11]. A large proportion of healthcare costs are spent on administration of insurers [12].

Americans with higher wages may get their insurance through their employers or privately. Figures show that employers with a high number of low paid employees are less likely to provide insurance benefits than those with a low number of low paid employees [13]. The Affordable Care Act (https://www.healthcare.gov/glossary/affordable-care-act/) has enabled those on low wage to get insurance or to shop around for insurance in the marketplace. However over the years the cost of healthcare and insurance premiums has increased. This is attributed to the longevity of the population and the increase in chronic debilitating diseases such as obesity and diabetes. This rising cost of healthcare quite often prohibits people from either not seeing a healthcare provider or delaying treatment or filling in a prescription. After the ACA, there still remains almost 32 million of the American population that remain uninsured [14].

This system it is claimed does not put the patient at the heart of the service. It is served to a large extent by insurers most of whom are for profit. Unnecessary tests are often done to avoid litigation, and the profits may be shared with the doctors.

The ethnic minorities, who live in the poorer neighbourhoods, have high mortality and morbidity. Visiting Atlanta, the home of Martin Luther King, the author (MK) found the town divided with the rich having access to a fully equipped private facility, and the ethnic minorities to a ill equipped hospital across the road, all in the same city.

How Can Governments Choose the Best Model of Healthcare?

Where governments have crumbled or the state infrastructure is in disarray, choosing the correct healthcare model can be difficult. Many a times, providing a healthcare model is superseded by political rivalry and infighting. Much less importance is given to considering the needs of the people, current cultural and structural organisations within the society at these times and more on delivering any 'model'. In 2002 in Afghanistan, a decision was made to privatise healthcare due to the preponderance of NGO's prevalent in the country with very little thought on building up the healthcare infrastructure from grass roots level [15]. It was felt that by providing such a model all the other problems would heal themselves. Similarity in Iraq, after the recent turmoil and change in government, there is very little progress in delivering a healthcare service for the people that meets the standards. Many hospitals remain in ruin, fully equipped but not operational or partially finished [16].

Conclusion

Healthcare is a basic right for all people globally. There remain vast differences in affordability of healthcare in the developed and developing world. Models vary from out of pocket, insured or government funded or a hybrid. Unfortunately vast numbers of people still do not have access to affordable healthcare and governments need to work hard to make this a priority.

References

1. Tax-based financing for health systems: options and experiences. Discussion paper number 4. 2004. Available at http://www.who.int/health_financing/taxed_based_financing_dp_04_4.pdf.
2. Reynolds E. Look at healthcare models around the world. Focus Economics; March 2018. Available at https://www.focus-economics.com/blog/a-look-at-healthcare-models-around-the-world.
3. Institute of Medicine (US) and National Academy of Engineering (US) Roundtable on Value & Science-Driven Health Care. Healthcare system complexities, impediments, and failures. In: Engineering a learning healthcare system: a look at the future: workshop summary. Washington, DC: National Academies Press; 2011. p. 117–70. Available from: https://www.ncbi.nlm.nih.gov/books/NBK61963/.
4. Massuda A, et al. The Brazilian health system at crossroads: progress, crisis and resilience. BMJ Glob Health. 2018;3(4):e000829.
5. Sawicki P, Bastian H. German healthcare: a bit of Bismarck plus more science. BMJ. 2008;337:a1997.
6. Chung M. Healthcare reform: learning from other major healthcare systems. Princeton Public Health Review. 2017. Available at https://pphr.princeton.edu/2017/12/02/unhealthy-health-care-a-cursory-overview-of-major-health-care-systems/.
7. Lorraine LS. A view of health care around the world. Ann Fam Med. 2013;11(1):84.
8. Lee SY, Chun CB, Lee YG, Seo NK. The National Health Insurance system as one type of new typology: the case of South Korea and Taiwan. Health Policy. 2008;85(1):105–13.
9. Anita J. Emerging health insurance in India - an overview. 10th Global Conference of Actuaries. https://www.actuariesindia.org/downloads/gcadata/10thGCA/Emerging%20Health%20Insurance%20in%20India-An%20overview_J%20Anitha.pdf.
10. Balch O. Indian law requires companies to give 2% of profits to charity. Is it working? The Guardian; 5 Apr 2016. Available at https://www.theguardian.com/sustainable-business/2016/apr/05/india-csr-law-requires-companies-profits-to-charity-is-it-working.
11. OECD. Health at a glance 2015. OECD Indicators. OECD Publishing; 2015. Available at http://www.oecd-ilibrary.org/social-issues-migration-health/health-at-a-glance_19991312.
12. Jiwani A, Himmelstein D, Woolhandler S, Kahn JG. Billing and insurance-related administrative costs

in United States' health care: synthesis of micro-costing evidence. BMC Health Serv Res. 2014;14:556. https://doi.org/10.1186/s12913-014-0556-7.

13. Long SH, Marquis MS. Low-wage workers and health insurance coverage: can policymakers target them through their employers? Inquiry. 2001;38(3):331–7.

14. Smith JC, Medalia C. Health insurance coverage in the United States: 2014. Current population reports.

U.S. Census Bureau. Washington, DC: Government Printing Office; 2015. p. 5.

15. Sabri B, Siddiqi S, Ahmed AM, Kakar FK, Perrot J. Towards sustainable delivery of health services in Afghanistan: options for the future. Bull World Health Organ. 2007;85(9):712–8.

16. Webster P. Reconstruction efforts in Iraq failing health care. Lancet. 2009;373(9664):617–20.

Part III

Provision of Effective, Safe and Good Quality Care

How Do Hospitals Deliver Safe, Effective and High Quality Care?

4

Patrick Dobbs

Over the years there have been several methods to assess whether care given in a hospital setting is safe. As healthcare scandals have occurred such as in Bristol paediatric heart surgery [1], or general care in Mid Staffordshire NHS Trust [2] both healthcare regulators and service providers have desired improved methodology to assess not only safety, but also the effectiveness and quality of care provided to patients and their families. This chapter will review how hospitals that are recognised for safe, effective and high quality care have done so, and how their lessons are shared to the wider healthcare community.

It is important to understand what the terms safe, effective and high quality mean in the context of a healthcare setting:

Safe Safe means that people are protected from abuse and avoidable harm (abuse can be physical, sexual, mental or psychological, financial, neglect, institutional or discriminatory abuse) [3]. Emphasis is placed on the system of care delivery that prevents errors; learns from the errors that do occur; and is built on a culture of safety that involves health care professionals, organizations, and patients [4].

Effective Effective means that people's care, treatment and support achieves good outcomes, promotes a good quality of life and is based on the best available evidence [3]. Effective also has meaning relating to how an organisation uses its resources to provide safe and effective care, the appropriate use of inputs (staff, equipment and medicines) at the lowest cost (economy) to achieve the best mix of high quality outputs (patients receiving treatment) [5].

High Quality Quality is a more nebulous concept in the healthcare setting in that it is the overarching feature that encompasses other indicators of care. The World Health Organisation (WHO) defines quality as: "the extent to which health care services provided to individuals and patient populations improve desired health outcomes. In order to achieve this, health care must be safe, effective, timely, efficient, equitable and people-centred" [6].

Combining the above definitions it can be considered that safe, effective and high quality care is when a patient receives the best evidenced treatment, without complications, efficiently through quicker recovery and shorter lengths of stay using appropriate resources.

Historically hospital safety was judged through crude markers such as mortality rates; these assumed homogeneity within healthcare organisations and could offer false assurance from favourable results. However variation in mortality

P. Dobbs (✉)
Sheffield Teaching Hospitals NHS Foundation Trust, Sheffield, UK
e-mail: Patrick.Dobbs@sth.nhs.uk

© Springer Nature Switzerland AG 2019
D. Burke et al. (eds.), *Hospital Transformation*, https://doi.org/10.1007/978-3-030-15448-6_4

rates cannot be ignored, as they might indicate unacceptable variation in healthcare and avoidable mortality, but they also cannot be reliably used to judge the quality of healthcare, based on current evidence [7]. This view was echoed by Sir Robert Francis "it is in my view misleading and a potential misuse of the figures to extrapolate from them a conclusion that any particular number, or range of numbers of deaths were caused or contributed to by inadequate care" [2].

Following the publication of Sir Bruce Keogh's report into care at 14 failing NHS trusts [8], the Care Quality Commission began examining in depth all NHS acute and specialist trusts across a range of metrics. This review summarised in the report "The state of care in NHS acute hospitals: 2014–2016" [3], is the most comprehensive examination of a healthcare system yet and is able to describe at service and organisational levels what safe, effective and high quality care looks like.

The CQC inspections involved a review of eight key services:

- Urgent and emergency services
- Medical care
- Surgery
- Critical care
- Maternity and gynaecology
- Services for children and young people
- End of life care
- Outpatients and diagnostic imaging

Each service was rated against the metrics of Safe, Effective, Caring, Responsive and Well Led, the ratings being on a four point scale, Outstanding, Good, Requires Improvement and Inadequate. These ratings are aggregated to provide an overall hospital rating as in Table 4.1.

The ratings provide a snapshot in time of the quality of care at core service, hospital and trust level [3].

It can be seen that the CQC inspections uncover variable practice within the same organisation, so even hospitals rated outstanding overall may have areas rated as requiring improvement.

The inspections when aggregated also provide new information regarding patient safety; Fig. 4.1 shows the relationship between CQC ratings and financial performance.

It can be deduced that hospitals rated as outstanding often do better financially than hospitals rated as providing at a lower level. The hypothesis for these findings is that hospitals that provide safe and effective care do not have the financial burden for prolonged lengths of stay and additional diagnostics, care and treatments when harm occurs.

The CQC inspections concluded that there was commonality between organisations that performed well, this can be summarised in Fig. 4.2.

In practice all six features are closely interrelated and each requires aspects of the others to succeed.

Table 4.1 An example of how the CQC rate a healthcare organisation

	Safe	Effective	Caring	Responsive	Well led	Overall
Urgent and emergency services	Good	Good	Good	Good	Good	Good
Medical care	Good	Good	Good	Good	Good	Good
Surgery	Good	Good	Good	Good	Good	Good
Critical care	Good	Outstanding	Good	Good	Outstanding	Outstanding
Maternity and gynaecology	Good	Good	Good	Outstanding	Outstanding	Outstanding
Services for children and young people	Good	Good	Good	Good	Good	Good
End of life care	Good	Requires improvement	Good	Good	Requires improvement	Requires improvement
Outpatients and diagnostic imaging	Good	Not rated	Good	Good	Outstanding	Outstanding
Overall	Good	Good	Good	Good	Outstanding	Good

Adapted CQC ratings for Sheffield Teaching Hospitals NHS Foundation Trust [9]

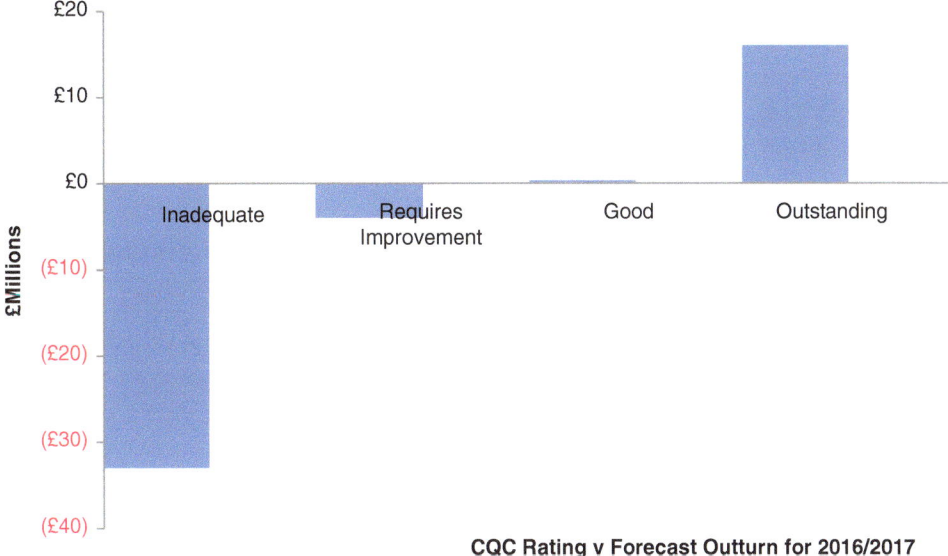

CQC Rating v Forecast Outturn for 2016/2017

Fig. 4.1 The relationship between CQC ratings and financial performance of Healthcare Organisations. Adapted from The State of Care In NHS Acute Hospitals 2014–2016 [3]

Fig. 4.2 Features of a high performing organisation

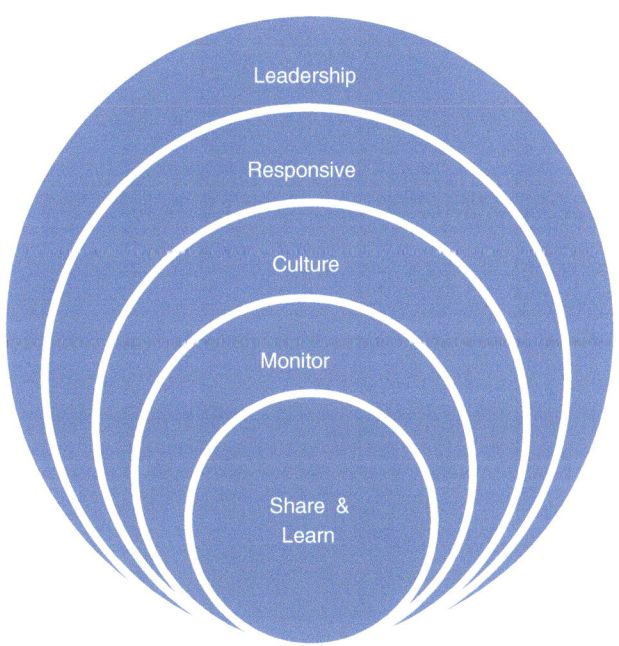

Leadership

It is clear that for an organisation to provide safe, effective and high quality care there must be effective and visible leadership throughout the organisation. This starts at board level, and con-

tinues to all levels of the organisation. The board is responsible for ensuring:

- The quality and safety of health services.
- That resources are invested in a way that delivers optimal health outcomes.

- In the accessibility and responsiveness of health services.
- That patients and the public can help to shape health services to meet their needs.
- That public money is spent in a way that is fair, efficient, effective and economic [10].

The CQC has found that in hospitals rated good or outstanding, the trust boards actively engaged with staff to determine how the organisation needed to improve. The composition and capabilities of the board have been shown to influence the ability of the board to engage with staff, and to encourage reporting and handling of patient safety issues [11]. Jones et al. state that boards with mature quality improvement (QI) cultures had strong clinical leadership and engaged staff and patients [12]. Moreover objective data presented to boards was enhanced by softer subjective data gleaned by clinical leaders from their encounters with staff in the clinical scenarios. These boards were also skilled in balancing short term external priorities with the needs of their own long term improvement initiatives [13]. There is increasing stress at executive level, with shorter tenures and increasing vacancies in trusts experiencing the most challenged levels of performance. Trusts rated as 'inadequate' by the Care Quality Commission had 14% of posts vacant, compared to only 3% in trusts rated as 'outstanding'. This has a knock on effect on staff who feel their leaders have less credibility, and also delays organisational progress [14]. Therefore consistent and lasting leadership at board level would seem important for an organisation to provide quality care.

Whilst leadership from the boards is essential, it is equally important that consistent leadership is in place at every level of the organisation. One reason given for the variability in quality within high performing organisations is poor leadership in certain areas. This leadership must be values-driven and coupled with a learning culture to provide high quality care [3].

Responsiveness

Responsiveness or agility in healthcare relates to the ability of an organisation to react and adapt quickly and successfully in the face of rapid change [15]. This may be in relation to a sudden influx of patients, changes in staff levels or national agenda items such as finance. Healthcare in general does not like change, and despite multiple efforts to improve, across the system there is inertia [16] and a reliance on previous experience to deal with times of stress.

Responsive health systems anticipate and adapt to changing needs, harness opportunities to promote access to effective interventions and improve quality of health services, ultimately leading to better health outcomes [17].

Responsiveness also means that services are organised to meet people's needs [18]:

- Services are planned for the population they serve;
- Care is coordinated with external agencies;
- Care is available when needed, without undue delay;
- Complaints and concerns are taken seriously and dealt with in a timely manner. Lessons are learnt from complaints

When services are designed to serve the population using them, they are more likely to provide a better patient experience which is associated with better health and financial outcomes [19].

Culture

Good leadership is the foundation for organisational culture. Baker [20] describes high performing international organisations whose leaders commit to building a professional culture that encourages improvement, patient engagement and teamwork. Organisations rated as outstanding by the CQC exhibited cultures that were open and honest, where staff were listened to about safety concerns and the board sought the views of patients and staff in ways in which the organisation could improve [3].

In Sir Robert Francis's review of creating an open and honest reporting culture within the NHS, Freedom to Speak Up [21] he defines what good looks like in a safe culture as:

- Culture of safety—a move away from blame to just, where safety questions are asked and addressed and learning gained from the process.
- Culture of raising concern—A shared belief at all levels of an organisation in speaking up about concerns, and supporting those who do so.
- Cultures free of bullying—bullying inhibits the freedom to speak up and is counter to the concept of a just culture.
- Culture of visible leadership—authenticity of leaders at all levels in espousing the values and beliefs of the organisation is paramount to the nurturing of a safety culture.
- Culture of valuing staff—recognising the value in raising concerns and supporting staff leads to better staff engagement. NHS staff surveys have shown improved staff engagement leads to better patient outcomes and financial performance.
- Culture of reflective practice—allowing staff to reflect on issues, systems and learning from incidents.

Staff engagement is a good mirror of the culture within an organisation and there is compelling evidence that quality of care, patient experience and mortality are directly related to staff engagement. Unfortunately the corollary of this is also true, where there is poor engagement, where staff do not feel valued, care suffers [22]. During the mid-2000's Mid Staffordshire NHS Foundation Trust had some of the lowest staff engagement scores in the NHS, a period associated with a lack of quality, safety and compassion. Conversely

Salford Royal NHS Foundation which has been rated as outstanding in successive CQC visits has some of the highest staff engagement scores. There is no magic bullet to improve culture and staff engagement. However having a set of core values and beliefs which put the patient first, are led by the board and practised by all staff would seem to be important. The King's Fund [23] has suggested six building blocks that over time will help to improve and harness staff engagement:

- Develop a compelling, shared strategic direction
- Build collective and distributed leadership
- Adopt supportive and inclusive leadership styles
- Give staff the tools to lead service transformation
- Establish a culture based on integrity and trust
- Place staff engagement firmly on the board agenda

The ultimate test of a vision has to be whether it transcends the mission statement and enters the organisation's bloodstream—the rites, rituals, cultural norms and stories about 'how we do things around here'. In November 2014, staff at Wrightington, Wigan and Leigh NHS Foundation Trust wheeled a 77-year-old cancer patient into the hospital car park to say goodbye to the horse she had cared for for more than 25 years. For staff, the message from the story is clear: this is an organisation that really is trying, as it claims in its mission statement, to put patients 'at the heart of everything we do', and is giving staff the freedom and support to translate the vision into practice.

Case Study adapted from the King's Fund [23].

Sustaining and embedding QI initiatives and staff involvement into the organisations culture can be problematic. Several organisations have adopted varying methods to ensure that initiatives become "business as usual". The following are examples from NHS Employers [24] where sustained improvement has become ingrained within the culture of the organisation:

Sheffield Teaching Hospitals

Developed a Micro Systems Coaching Academy to support staff to improve in their workplace. The aims of the academy are:

- Build improvement capability into the workforce
- Maximise quality and value to patients
- Help multi-disciplinary front-line teams rethink and redesign services.

The teams are coached by staff trained in service improvement methodology to redesign their services.

Tees Esk and Wear Valley

This is a specialist mental health organisation and has a longstanding commitment to staff engagement and service improvement. It started out with a focus on Lean methods. It has a large number of staff trained in using quality improvement tools, and recently it has developed a local quality improvement system (QIS), which emphasises that staff know best. The aim of the QIS is to:

- Analyse existing practice
- Enable staff to determine what is changed and how
- Provide staff with tools to make change.

Ashford and St Peter's Hospitals NHS Foundation Trust

Be the Change programme was initially developed by junior doctors. The trust focussed on involving as many staff as possible in making small improvements in their own areas, with the aim being to build up a culture of improvement. It provided:

- The opportunity to share ideas for improvement
- The opportunity for frontline staff to become change champions
- Developmental opportunities.

Hundreds of postcards were submitted with ideas for improvement, and over 40 quality improvement projects were launched with a junior doctor and change champion leading each one. The top three projects received recognition by the executive team and support to full implementation. These and others examples demonstrate sustained quality improvement that becomes ingrained to the organisational culture.

Monitor

For an organisation to know it is safe and provides quality care it needs to measure and analyse its performance. It has already been stated that simple measures of an organisation such as mortality rates are crude and insufficient. So what should an organisation measure and monitor?

External inspections, such as those by the CQC provide a snapshot in time, but are an indication of how the organisation performs against a fundamental set of standards of safety and quality [25]. A high quality organisation must continuously monitor and learn to ensure patient safety and compassionate care. However in 2013 Berwick found "that most healthcare organisations at present have very little capacity to analyse, monitor or learn from safety and quality information" [26].

One approach developed in the UK was to design a framework for safety encompassing five domains [27]:

- Have we been safe in the past?
- Are systems and processes reliable?
- Is care safe today?

- Will care be safe in the future?
- Are we responding and improving?

This approach allows an organisation to assess and reflect on its past, present and future ability to provide quality care at organisational level. It relies on the ability to measure various indicators in each domain; however this can be problematic as most organisations do not collect the required data in a meaningful way. Furthermore NHS Trusts often rely on too few metrics to assure themselves on the quality of their services [3].

Another approach gaining acceptance in the US and some European countries is to monitor what matters to the patient, based on the values based healthcare delivery (VBHCD) described by Porter [28]. In this methodology there is recognition that existing monitoring is generally of process compliance with guidelines or headline values such as mortality rather than the patient's experience. In contrast VBHCD measures outcomes across three tiers, specific to the disease or intervention at a patient level. For example below would be the outcomes for a hip replacement operation:

- Tier 1
  - Health Status achieved or retained
    - Survival (eg Mortality)
  - Degree of health or Recovery
    - Functional level achieved
    - Pain level achieved
    - Ability to return to work
- Tier 2
  - Process of recovery
    - Time to begin treatment
    - Time to return to physical activities
    - Time to return to work
  - Disutility of care or treatment process (eg diagnostic errors, ineffective care, complications, adverse effects)
    - Delays and anxiety
    - Pain during treatment
    - Length of hospital stay
    - Infection
    - Venous thromboembolism/ Myocardial infarction
    - Need for re-operation

- Tier 3 Sustainability of health
  - Nature of recurrences
    - Maintained functional level
    - Ability to live independently
    - Need for revision or replacement
  - Long term consequences of therapy
    - Loss of mobility due to inadequate rehabilitation
    - Susceptibility to infection
    - Regional pain

Adapted from Measuring Health Outcomes Michael Porter New England Journal of Medicine [29].

These outcomes can be compared locally, nationally or internationally as a driver for quality improvement.

Outcomes measurement has become a science in itself, national and international cooperation is required in order that consistent and comprehensive measurement is achieved globally.

This methodology will allow meaningful comparison to occur and rapid improvement be stimulated.

An international group has been established to develop and publish agreed outcome measurements, the International Consortium for Health Outcomes Measurement (ICHOM) [30].

However data is collected, it is clear that to provide high quality and safe healthcare an organisation must devote resource to continually monitoring and reacting to the services it provides. Using benchmarking in an open and transparent fashion against similar organisations locally, nationally and internationally can only drive up quality.

Sharing and Learning

One of the factors that differentiated hospitals rated as outstanding by the CQC from those rated as inadequate was the culture around how the hospitals dealt with safety concerns [3]. Unsurprisingly it appears that an organisation which listens to its staff, has an open and learning culture and learns from issues raised will provide better care to the population it serves. Authenticity in organisational values and behaviours is critically important in developing this culture. In the NHS all staff have a duty to protect patients from harm [31], however staff may be inhibited from doing so if a blame culture exists. In addition some hospitals use incident reporting as a performance management tool which leads to investigation fatigue and overload of the systems, potentially leading to missed opportunities to learn from patient safety issues [32]. All NHS organisations must have a system for reporting near misses and harm, and should examine and assess if any learning should be gleaned from incidents. In addition in England and Wales there has existed since 2003, a National Reporting and Learning System (NRLS), which is a central database of patient safety incident reports. All information submitted is analysed to identify hazards, risks and opportunities to continuously improve the safety of patient care [33]. Information is passed back to all organisations in a monthly report to disseminate.

Italy has a relatively recent safety policy agenda; set up in 2008 the National Observatory on Good Practices for Patient Safety it is regarded as a model for international health organisations to emulate [25].

> The National Observatory on Good Practices for Patient Safety is designed to:
>
> • Address the heterogeneity of care across Italy's 21 regional healthcare systems in relation to patient safety issues.
> • Identify and disseminate good practice to reduce poor health outcomes
> • Evaluate implementation of good practice and respond to the feedback from the healthcare systems
> • Understand the barriers for implementation
> • Monitor compliance using questionnaires
> • Promote ownership among professionals and healthcare systems (including patients and citizens).

> By utilising improvement methodology (PDSA cycles) and a bi-directional approach the National Observatory has succeeded in implementing a national patient safety initiative that can be transferable across national and international healthcare systems.

Case study on National Observatory on Good Practices [25, 34].

Conclusions

No one hospital or organisation will have all the answers to providing the best quality, safe and effective care for the populations it serves. However the hospitals rated highest will have, to some extent, aspects of all the above factors ingrained into the way they operate. The challenges lying ahead of reduced staff levels (especially nursing), junior doctor's numbers and training, and the implications for BREXIT on the NHS will severely test the ability of organisations to function. Those who demonstrate the values espoused above have a greater chance of continuing to serve their patients with compassion in a safe and engaged environment.

References

1. Teasdale GM. Learning from Bristol: report of the public inquiry into children's heart surgery at Bristol Royal Infirmary 1984-1995. Br J Neurosurg. 2002;16(3):211–6.
2. Francis R. Report of the mid staffordshire NHS foundation trust public inquiry. New directions for youth development. London: The Stationery Office; 2013.
3. The state of care in NHS acute hospitals [Internet] [cited 2018 Sep 17]. Available from: https://www.cqc.org.uk/sites/default/files/20170302b_stateofhospitals_web.pdf.
4. Barton A. Patient safety and quality: an evidence-based handbook for nurses. AORN J. 2009; 90(4):601–2.
5. Delivering cost effective care in the NHS [Internet] [cited 2018 Sep 17]. Available from: https://www.cqc.

org.uk/sites/default/files/20151028_delivering_cost_effective_care_in_the_NHS.pdf.

6. WHO. What is quality of care and why is it important? [Internet]. World Health Organization; 2017 [cited 2018 Sep 17]. p. 1–4. Available from: http://www.who.int/maternal_child_adolescent/topics/quality-of-care/definition/en/.

7. Goodacre S, Campbell M, Carter A. What do hospital mortality rates tell us about quality of care? Emerg Med J [Internet]. 2015 Mar 1 [cited 2018 Sep 17];32(3):244–7. Available from: http://www.ncbi.nlm.nih.gov/pubmed/24064042.

8. Keogh B. Review into the quality of care and treatment provided by 14 hospital trusts in England: overview report. London: Hm Govt; 2013.

9. Care Quality Commission. Sheffield Teaching Hospitals NHS Foundation Trust quality report [Internet]. 2016 [cited 2018 Sep 17]. Available from: https://www.cqc.org.uk/sites/default/files/new_reports/AAAE8129.pdf.

10. Bennett D, Flory D. The healthy NHS board [Internet]. 2013. Available from: www.foresight-partnership.co.uk.

11. Mannion R, Davies HTO, Jacobs R, Kasteridis P, Millar R, Freeman T. Do hospital boards matter for better, safer, patient care? Soc Sci Med [Internet]. 2017 Mar;177:278–87. Available from: https://www.sciencedirect.com/science/article/pii/S0277953617300527.

12. Jones L, Pomeroy L, Robert G, Burnett S, Anderson JE, Fulop NJ. How do hospital boards govern for quality improvement? A mixed methods study of 15 organisations in England. BMJ Qual Saf [Internet]. 2017 Dec;26(12):978–86. Available from: http://www.ncbi.nlm.nih.gov/pubmed/28689191.

13. Alderwick H, Charles A, Jones B, Warburton W. Making the case for quality improvement: lessons for NHS boards and leaders. London: The Kings Fund; 2017. https://www.kingsfund.org.uk/publications/making-case-quality-improvement.

14. Anandaciva S, Ward D, Randhawa M, Edge R. Leadership in today's NHS. The King's Fund [Internet]. [cited 2018 Sep 12]. Available from: https://www.kingsfund.org.uk/publications/leadership-todays-nhs.

15. Why agility is imperative for healthcare organizations. McKinsey on Healthcare [Internet]. [cited 2018 Sep 17]. Available from: https://healthcare.mckinsey.com/why-agility-imperative-healthcare-organizations.

16. Braithwaite J. Changing how we think about healthcare improvement. BMJ [Internet]. 2018 May 17 [cited 2018 Sep 12];361:k2014. Available from: http://www.ncbi.nlm.nih.gov/pubmed/29773537.

17. Tolib Mirzoev SK. What is health systems responsiveness? Review of existing knowledge and proposed conceptual framework. [cited 2018 Sep 18]; Available from: http://resyst.lshtm.ac.uk/.

18. CQC. How CQC regulates: NHS and independent acute hospitals. Provider handbook, March 2015 [Internet]. 2015 [cited 2018 Sep 12]. Available from: https://www.cqc.org.uk/sites/default/files/20150327_acute_hospital_provider_handbook_march_15_update_01.pdf.

19. Churchill N. Domain 4: ensuring that people have a positive experience of care [Internet]. 2013 [cited 2018 Sep 18]. Available from: https://www.england.nhs.uk/wp-content/uploads/2013/11/pat-expe.pdf.

20. Baker GR (Commission on L, in the Nhs) M. The roles of leaders in high-performing health care systems. Comm Leadersh Manag NHS Kings Fund. 2011.

21. Freedom to speak up an independent review into creating an open and honest reporting culture in the NHS Freedom to speak up-a review of whistleblowing in the NHS 2 [Internet]. 2015 [cited 2018 Sep 11]. Available from: http://freedomtospeakup.org.uk/wp-content/uploads/2014/07/F2SU_web.pdf.

22. Ham C. Improving NHS care by engaging staff and devolving decision making: report of the review of staff engagement and empowerment in the NHS. King's Fund [Internet]. 2014 [cited 2018 Sep 11];2014:1–76. Available from: https://www.kingsfund.org.uk/sites/default/files/field/field_publication_file/improving-nhs-care-by-engaging-staff-and-devolving-decision-making-jul14.pdf.

23. Collins B. Staff engagement Six building blocks for harnessing the creativity and enthusiasm of NHS staff [Internet]. 2015 [cited 2018 Sep 11]. Available from: https://www.kingsfund.org.uk/sites/default/files/field/field_publication_file/staff-engagement-feb-2015.pdf.

24. NHSEmployers. Staff involvement, quality improvement and staff engagement. The missing links? Brief 110 [Internet]. 2017 [cited 2018 Sep 11];(July). Available from: http://www.nhsemployers.org/-/media/Employers/Publications/Staff-involvement-quality-improvement-and-staff-engagement.pdf.

25. Caring for quality in health lessons learnt from 15 reviews of health care quality [Internet]. [cited 2018 Sep 11] Available from: https://www.oecd.org/els/health-systems/Caring-for-Quality-in-Health-Final-report.pdf.

26. Department of Health. A promise to learn-a commitment to act: improving the safety of patients in England. National Advisory Group on the Safety of Patients in England [Internet]. 2013 [cited 2018 Sep 11]. Available from: https://assets.publishing.service.gov.uk/government/uploads/system/uploads/attachment_data/file/226703/Berwick_Report.pdf.

27. Vincent C, Burnett S, Carthey J. Safety measurement and monitoring in healthcare: a framework to guide clinical teams and healthcare organisations in maintaining safety. BMJ Qual Saf [Internet]. 2014 Aug 1 [cited 2018 Sep 11];23(8):670–7. Available from: http://www.ncbi.nlm.nih.gov/pubmed/24764136.

28. Harvard Business School. Value-based health care delivery - institute for strategy and competitiveness - Harvard Business School [Internet]. 2014 [cited 2018 Sep 11]. p. 1. Available from: https://www.isc.hbs.edu/health-care/vbhcd/Pages/default.aspx.

29. Porter ME. What is value in health care? N Engl J Med [Internet]. 2010 Dec 23 [cited 2018 Sep 11];363(26):2477–81. Available from: http://www.nejm.org/doi/abs/10.1056/NEJMp1011024.

30. ICHOM – international consortium for health outcomes measurement [Internet]. [cited 2018 Sep 17]. Available from: http://www.ichom.org/.

31. Openness and honesty when things go wrong: the professional duty of candour [Internet]. [cited 2018 Sep 17]. Available from: www.nmc.org.uk/concerns-nurses-midwives/.

32. NHS Improvement: "investigation fatigue" prevents trusts learning from mistakes. Health Serv J [Internet]. [cited 2018 Sep 17]. Available from: https://www.hsj.co.uk/policy-and-regulation/nhs-improvement-investigation-fatigue-prevents-trusts-learning-from-mistakes/7021967.article.

33. NRLS reporting [Internet]. [cited 2018 Sep 17]. Available from: https://report.nrls.nhs.uk/nrlsreporting/.

34. Labella B, Giannantoni P, Raho V, Tozzi Q, Caracci G. Disseminating good practices for patient safety: the experience of the Italian National Observatory on Good Practices for Patient Safety. Epidemiol Biostat Public Health. 2016 [cited 2018 Dec 21]. Available from: https://ebph.it/article/download/11691/10842.

Part IV

Identifying Failure

Stephen Duckett and Christine Jorm

Accreditation plays an important role in regulatory oversight of hospitals and other health care institutions in most advanced economies. Although accreditation started as a voluntary process, it has evolved in many countries to be effectively compulsory [1]. The formula for accreditation is common, possibly driven by the influence of the international organisation, the International Society for Quality in Health Care (ISQua) which accredits the accreditors. The formula involves:

- Published standards;
- Hospital visits by 'surveyors' to assess the hospital against the standards; and
- A decision to 'accredit' or not.

The standards generally apply to all organisations seeking accreditation with little adaption to the specific circumstances or performance of an individual organization. The same questions about infection control, for example, are asked in a hospital which has the best performance on hospital acquired infections, as in the worst performer.

S. Duckett (✉)
Grattan Institute, Carlton, VIC, Australia
e-mail: stephen.duckett@grattan.edu.au

C. Jorm
NSW Regional Health Partners,
Newcastle, NSW, Australia
e-mail: Christine.jorm@health.nsw.gov.au

Although accreditation has been around for almost a century [2], the tried and true formula is under challenge. Participation in accreditation is a time consuming and expensive exercise yet the overall value of accreditation is unclear. The current approach emphasises accountability and assurance rather than improvement, alienating many clinicians: when it ignores their priorities, they dismiss it as irrelevant [3].

Accreditation is failing and needs to be transformed. In this chapter we describe a transformation path.

Data Driven Improvement

The main focus of accreditation has been on structures surrounding care (process measures), even though the early twentieth century US surgeon whose work stimulated hospital accreditation, Ernest Codman, designed an 'end results system' [4, 5], what we today would describe as an outcomes focus.

Accreditation has not kept pace with the dramatic improvement that has occurred in hospital outcomes measurement in recent decades. There is now a wealth of data collected on patient care, including most importantly, information on whether diagnoses were present on admission or arose during the course of the admission [6, 7], the latter can legitimately be described as complications of care. Routine data, adequately risk-adjusted, is now in widespread use in many countries to compare hospital performance [8].

Traditional accreditation has not adapted to this improvement in the ability to measure hospital performance. Routine data can be used to measure the rarely occurring sentinel events [9], as well as more frequently occurring complications such as hospital-acquired infections [10]. Although these data are not perfect [11], and generally cannot be used to identify complications which are always preventable, they can be used to identify comparative performance of hospitals [12]. By comparing rates of total complications, whether those complications can be labelled preventable or not, differences in rates between the best and worst hospitals can be used to identify opportunities for improvement—when the best performing hospitals are identified, other institutions can learn from them [13].

The key transformation required for hospital accreditation is to shift from assessment of generic one-size-fits-all process-centred standards to a targeted, hospital-specific approach which is data driven. Accreditation should focus on each hospital's specific issues in a structured and transparent way, to help it hospital respond to improvement opportunities.

Types of Regulation

Organisations respond to incentives [14]. In health care, what is regulated shapes what hospitals give priority to:

In healthcare systems, the impetus for change can vary from subtle to strident; it can be founded on fear or on hope; built on pressure to conform or an imperative to be distinguished; adopt an attitude of support or challenge; can be tacit or codified; and focused or pervasive in scope. Pressure to change can come from within or from outside—inducements can take the form of hugs, nudges or shoves [15].

Healthcare regulation conveys messages about what issues are important and how important they are. There are many regulators and regulatory mechanisms. Design of regulation often seeks to ensure that it is risk-based and responsive.

Risk-based regulation focuses on the highest-priority risks, determined by assessment of their probability and consequences [16]. There is no attempt to prevent all possible harms. Ideally, low-risk providers are free from the burden of inspection, and inspectors concentrate on organisations with poor practice. Effective regulation thus controls risk while identifying important problems and solving them [17–19].

Responsive regulation assumes the parties being regulated are trust-worthy and intrinsically motivated [19]. Most effort is therefore put into encouraging co-operation (through persuasion) rather than enforcing compliance. However, a range of enforcement measures of graduated severity must be available ('the regulatory pyramid').

Really responsive regulation holds that sensitivity to change is central to regulatory performance:

If regulators cannot adapt to change, they will apply yesterday's controls to today's problems and … under-performance will be in-evitable [20].

The emphasis of this approach is on changing measures in response to organisational performance. Timely feedback and use of contemporary data means it also allows assessment of the value of the regulation itself:

If regulators cannot assess the performance of their regimes, they cannot know whether their efforts (and budgets) are having any positive effect in furthering their objectives. Nor can they justify their operations to the outside world [20].

A new system of accreditation should be *really responsive*: it needs to adapt to the overall changed measurement environment discussed above, the performance of each institution accredited and it also needs to build on and reinforce hospitals' and clinicians' intrinsic motivation to improve their safety performance.

Problems with Current Hospital Accreditation Systems

Wide variation in complication rates between hospitals observed in most countries suggests the accreditation systems have failed [21]. Practically every significant safety failure in Australia in recent decades has occurred in a hospital which had passed accreditation with flying colours, and the same is true in many other countries.

Problems with the current accreditation systems have been known for decades, despite regular attempts to improve their effectiveness. What little literature there is provides inconsistent and unconvincing evidence for the value of accreditation for improving the quality and safety of patient care [22–26]. Only one paper has explicitly sought to explore the potential mechanisms of impact of accreditation [3].

Denmark recently introduced accreditation and then rapidly discontinued it for public hospitals after claims by doctors and nurses that they were 'drowning in manuals and paperwork and have no time for patients' [27]. Denmark now uses a quality assurance model, based on high-levels of compliance with clinical quality registries, using those registries to monitor and improve quality [28].

As part of the accreditation process, hospitals compile evidence—such as policy documents, committee minutes, training documents and audit results—to show they are meeting the relevant standards. Auditors (or 'surveyors') assess a hospital's performance during an accreditation visit, which in Australia is up to 5 days. They examine documents and interview staff. Auditors may also observe clinical practice and inspect resources, such as signage and personal protective equipment, but they have limited time available to do this [29].

An accreditation visit itself results in a period of abnormal care. US research suggests hospitals may improve their performance during accreditation visits. One study showed significantly lower '30-day mortality' for patients admitted during the week of an unannounced accreditation visit than patients admitted in the 3 weeks before or after the visit [30]. Yet the aim of accreditation should be to encourage improved outcomes for patients admitted every week of the year.

The nature and subject of standards is central to accreditation—they communicate what the regulator thinks is important. There is little evidence examining the development, writing, implementation and impacts of healthcare accreditation standards [31].

The standards should be linked to important patient outcomes, and unfortunately many current indicators have no clear, evidence-based link to patient outcomes [32]. As healthcare is continually changing, indicators should be re-evaluated regularly, including by establishing and reassessing links to important patient outcomes, and assessing the experience in the best hospitals, which can be used as benchmarks. The decision can then be made to 'retain, revise, replace, or retire' them [32]. If links to important outcomes were not clear when standards were developed it becomes hard to reassess their utility. However, clear and direct links to important outcomes are not apparent in many current standards.

Another problem with most sets of standards is that while each individual standard may be intrinsically 'worthy', the set do not represent measured solutions proportionate in size to measured patient harms. Correcting this would require a comprehensive approach to patient outcomes, considering what improvements are possible, based on the best institutions [13]. Cost should also be considered: some areas will represent better investments than others. Understanding the cost of complications can also help in ensuring appropriate attention to frequently occurring harms, compared to the rare but dramatic adverse event [33].

Another problem with accreditation is that there are doubts about the validity and reliability of surveyor-based assessments, because different surveyors provide different opinions [34, 35].

Reviews consistently demonstrate doctors' scepticism about accreditation systems [22]. Doctors are concerned about the cost of accreditation programs, their bureaucratic and prescriptive nature, and the demands made on staff, and they believe these programs have no impact on the quality of care. They may feel accountable to themselves, their peers, and their profession, but not to accreditation bodies [36, 37]. The evidence shows doctors do not 'buy-in' to the accreditation process [38].

Additionally, in Australia at least, accreditors mostly assess work 'as imagined', or as described in the ideal case; they do not assess management of high-risk situations [29, 39]. This approach in England has resulted in criticism of accreditation for failing to focus on 'real achievements and outcomes for patients', and because of this it has been identified as contributing to a major hospital quality scandal [40].

A New Model for Accreditation

The failures of the current system are manifold. Radical change is needed.

Accreditation needs to move from being an 'event' in a hospital's calendar, to being a tool for a hospital's continuous improvement. The emphasis should move from compliance to improvement, and from qualitative assessments against standards to being based on measurable change in terms of key dimensions of quality. The accreditation process itself should be more accountable through transparency about who is doing the accreditation survey and what assessments are being made.

Consistent with a *really responsive* approach to regulation, hospital accreditation should be reoriented to focus on helping hospitals improve, rather than simply judging them against 'standards'. Responsibility for improving hospital safety should be local, clinically-led and overseen by each hospital's governance processes, with the accreditation process supporting and assessing a hospital's progress in addressing the hospital's specific safety issues as measured in the data. We propose five strategies to encourage a tailored, improvement-focused approach:

1. Comparative data about each hospital's performance should be provided to the hospital at least yearly. The data needs to be clinically relevant and sufficiently detailed to allow hospitals to drill down to clinical unit level [11, 41]. Who should provide the data will vary by country: it may be a hospital regulatory body,

Table 5.1 Measures to be used in new accreditation processes

Measure	Advantages
Clinical outcome measures—with an initial focus on hospital acquired complications (later others measures such as Patient Reported Outcome Measures could be added)	These are important objective measures (and there is no dispute about their value as occurs with process indicators)
Patient experience measures	There is strong evidence linking staff and patient experience to clinical outcomes. These measures are relevant to all patient outcomes and harms (not just a selection). For more detail see Duckett et al. [42]
Staff experience measures	

the funder in a public system, or private benchmarking groups.

The data should measure three things: clinical outcomes (at first focusing on hospital-acquired complications but later adding other outcomes, including patient-reported outcomes); patients' experiences; and staff members' experiences. The advantages of each of the three measures are set out in Table 5.1.

2. Each hospital and clinical unit should develop an improvement plan based on its own contemporary data.

3. Progress against this plan should be checked at least once a year by external accreditors.

4. Surveyors should spend a day reviewing the data and plan, and then a day meeting with the Board and senior management. These meetings should focus on assisting the hospital's own improvement efforts. The whole process should be about improvement, not blame [43].

5. Surveyor assessments of each hospital and specialty, together with quantitative data such as complication rates, should be made publicly available. Surveyors should be publicly identified, just as journal reviewers are increasingly expected to be. This would ensure they are publicly accountable for their conclusions

A New Approach to Safety Assurance

A safety regulatory system should not be solely about improvement—safety assurance is still important. However, in a new model, hospitals should self-certify for a set of basic standards, or 'process measures', with no evidence of audit required. This would reduce paperwork and free-up independent accreditors to test safety and to support hospitals' improvement activities. (These basic standards themselves could occasionally be audited using a risk-based approach.)

Auditors should make unannounced or short-notice visits to check on problems or high-risk situations recently identified elsewhere in the state or nation. These hospital visits would *not* be about compliance with traditional accreditation standards, but about testing safety as is in real-life practice in the hospital. It still may involve data, for example, by using evidence about hospital acquired infections reported in routine data as part of judging whether infection control systems are working in practice.

Table 5.2 Why transformed accreditation is better than the current model

Problem with current model	Advantage of new model
There is a lack of evidence that it improves patient outcomes	New data sources and improvement plans will help accreditation 'work'
Standards lack a strong evidence base	Major emphasis on patient outcomes, patient experience and staff experience replaces process-based standards—all have solid evidence
Different surveyors use different methods	Comprehensive objective data will be used
Medical staff are not engaged in the process	The focus on patient outcomes, and the potential consequences for poor performance, will ensure staff are engaged
Patient outcomes are not systematically measured, and safety is not tested	Patient outcomes will be measured, and safety will be tested during unannounced visits
There are no incentives for excellence	The publication of unit-level results will encourage excellence
Accreditation results are either not made public or are difficult to find	Detailed accreditation results will be readily available to the public

The Implications of the New Model

Our new model is radically different from current accreditation processes internationally.

Hospital accreditation schemes cost money—both in terms of direct outlays on fees and preparation time, but also in terms of time spent by managers and clinicians preparing for accreditation which would be better spent on other quality improvement activities. Poor quality care also costs money, in addition to causing harm [33, 44–46]. Therefore a better accreditation scheme should be seen as an investment to improve the quality of care and reduce the costs of poor quality.

Table 5.2 summarises the benefits of our new model of accreditation.

Conclusion

Hospital accreditation internationally requires a major overhaul. The current system has proven ineffective and modifications to it won't produce the systematic attention to patient outcomes we need. Our proposed new model replaces a focus on processes and compliance with minimum standards with a focus on local patient outcomes and improvement. Meaningful local outcomes will engage clinicians.

Hospitals will no longer be spruced up for an infrequent planned 'big event' accreditation visit. Instead, surveyors will conduct safety tests without notice and provide scrutiny and support for hospital's improvement work. Attention to the operation of a continuous outcomes-data based improvement plan becomes the major role of the hospital board. We believe that this proposal will create a systematic approach to reducing the incidence of all harms to hospital patients and therefore to reducing the cost of complications.

References

1. Shaw CD, et al. Profiling health-care accreditation organizations: an international survey. Int J Qual Health Care. 2013;25(3):222–31.
2. Joint Commission on Accreditation of Healthcare Organizations, editor. A study in hospital efficiency: as demonstrated by the case report of the first five years of a private hospital by E.A. Codman, MD. Illinois: Joint Commission; 1996.
3. Desveaux L, et al. Understanding the impact of accreditation on quality in healthcare: a grounded theory approach. Int J Qual Health Care. 2017;29(7):941–7.
4. Donabedian A. The end results of health care: Ernest Codman's contribution to quality assessment and beyond. Milbank Q. 1989;67(2):233–56.
5. Neuhauser D. Ernest Amory Codman, MD, and end results of medical care. Int J Technol Assess Health Care. 1990;6(2):307–25.
6. Glance LG, et al. Does date stamping ICD-9-CM codes increase the value of clinical information in administrative data? Health Serv Res. 2006;41(1):231–51.
7. Jackson TJ, et al. Development of a validation algorithm for 'present on admission' flagging. BMC Med Inform Decis Mak. 2009;9:48.
8. Organisation for Economic Cooperation and Development. Tackling wasteful spending on health. Paris: OECD; 2017.
9. Jackson TJ, et al. Monitoring sentinel events using routine inpatient data. Asia Pac J Health Manag. 2009;4(2):34–40.
10. Jackson TJ, et al. A classification of hospital-acquired diagnoses for use with routine hospital data. Med J Aust. 2009;191(10):544–8.
11. Duckett S, Jorm C, Danks L. Strengthening safety statistics: how to make hospital safety data more useful. Melbourne: Grattan Institute; 2017.
12. Duckett S, et al. All complications should count: using our data to make hospitals safer. Melbourne: Grattan Institute; 2018.
13. Hollnagel E. Safety-I and safety-II: the past and future of safety management. Farnham: Ashgate Publishing Company; 2014.
14. Frølich A, et al. A behavioral model of clinician responses to incentives to improve quality. Health Policy. 2007;80(1):179–93.
15. Levesque J-F, Sutherland K. What role does performance information play in securing improvement in healthcare? A conceptual framework for levers of change. BMJ Open. 2017;7(8):e014825.
16. Beaussier A-L, et al. Accounting for failure: risk-based regulation and the problems of ensuring healthcare quality in the NHS. Health Risk Soc. 2016;18(3–4):205–24.
17. Braithwaite J, Makkai T, Braithwaite V. Regulating aged care: ritualism and the new pyramid. Northampton, MA: Edward Elgar; 2007.
18. Drahos P, editor. Regulatory theory: foundations and applications. Acton: ANU Press; 2017.
19. Healy J, Braithwaite J. Designing safer health care through responsive regulation. Med J Aust. 2006;184(10 Suppl):S56–9.
20. Black J, Baldwin R. Really responsive risk-based regulation. Law Policy. 2010;32(2):181–213.
21. Griffith JR. Is it time to abandon hospital accreditation? Am J Med Qual. 2018;33(1):30–6.
22. Alkhenizan A, Shaw C. Impact of accreditation on the quality of healthcare services: a systematic review of the literature. Ann Saudi Med. 2011;31(4):407–16.
23. Bogh SB, et al. Improvement in quality of hospital care during accreditation: a nationwide stepped-wedge study. Int J Qual Health Care. 2016;28(6):715–20.
24. Brubakk K, et al. A systematic review of hospital accreditation: the challenges of measuring complex intervention effects. BMC Health Serv Res. 2015;15(1):1–10.
25. Greenfield D, et al. Health service accreditation reinforces a mindset of high-performance human resource management: lessons from an Australian study. Int J Qual Health Care. 2014;26(4):372–7.
26. Hinchcliff R, et al. Short-notice and unannounced survey methods: literature review. Sydney: Australian Commission on Safety and Quality in Health Care; 2017.
27. Denmark. Ministeriet for Sundhed og Forebyggelse. Sundhedsministeren og regionerne vil have mere kvalitet og mindre bureaukrati. Copenhagen; 2015.
28. Denmark.Sundhedsdatastyrelsen. Bekendtgørelse om godkendelse af landsdækkende og regionale kliniske kvalitetsdatabaser. Copenhagen; 2016.
29. Daly M, et al. Much to learn: lessons from other industries for healthcare accreditation. In: ISQua: learning at the system level to improve healthcare quality and safety. London: ISQua; 2017.
30. Barnett ML, Olenski AR, Jena AB. Patient mortality during unannounced accreditation surveys at us hospitals. JAMA Intern Med. 2017;177(5):693–700.
31. Greenfield D, et al. The standard of healthcare accreditation standards: a review of empirical research underpinning their development and impact. BMC Health Serv Res. 2012;12(1):1–14.
32. Chazapis M, et al. Perioperative structure and process quality and safety indicators: a systematic review. Br J Anaesth. 2018;120(1):51–66.
33. Jackson TJ, et al. Marginal costs of hospital-acquired conditions: information for priority-setting for patient

safety programmes and research. J Health Serv Res Policy. 2011;16(3):141–6.

34. Greenfield D, et al. The impact of national accreditation reform on survey reliability: a 2-year investigation of survey coordinators' perspectives. J Eval Clin Pract. 2016;22(5):662–7.

35. Newman S. Language-games and quality improvement in healthcare in England. Open Med J. 2017;4(1):73–85.

36. Jorm C. Reconstructing medical practice: engagement, professionalism and critical relationships in health care. Farnham: Gower; 2012.

37. Stoelwinder J, McNeil JJ, Ibrahim JA. A study of doctors' views on how hospital accreditation can assist them provide quality and safe care to consumers. Melbourne: Monash University, Department of Epidemiology and Preventive Medicine; 2004.

38. Pannick S, Sevdalis N, Athanasiou T. Beyond clinical engagement: a pragmatic model for quality improvement interventions, aligning clinical and managerial priorities. BMJ Qualit Saf. 2016;25(9):716–25.

39. Chatburn E, Macrae C, Carthey J, Vincent C. Measurement and monitoring of safety: impact and challenges of putting a conceptual framework into practice. BMJ Qual Saf. 2018;27(10):818–26.

40. Mid Staffordshire NHS Foundation Trust Public Inquiry (Chair: Robert Francis). Report. London: The Stationery Office; 2013.

41. MacLean CH, Kerr EA, Qaseem A. Time out - charting a path for improving performance measurement. N Engl J Med. 2018;378(19):1757–61.

42. Duckett S, et al. Safer care saves money: how to improve patient care and save public money at the same time. Melbourne: Grattan Institute; 2018.

43. Armstrong N, et al. Taking the heat or taking the temperature? A qualitative study of a large-scale exercise in seeking to measure for improvement, not blame. Soc Sci Med. 2018;198:157–64.

44. Ehsani J, Jackson T, Duckett S. The incidence and cost of adverse events in Victorian hospitals 2003-04. MJA. 2006;184(11):551–5.

45. Jackson TJ. One dollar in seven: scoping the economics of patient safety. Edmonton: Canadian Patient Safety Institute; 2009.

46. McNair P, Jackson T, Borovnicar D. Public hospital admissions for treating complications of clinical care: incidence, costs and funding strategy. Aust N Z J Public Health. 2010;34(3):330–3.

Key Features in Identifying Failing Hospitals

Rivanna Stuhler and Martin A. Koyle

Introduction

Hospitals, unlike other large institutions such as those in business or industry, are complex organizations, operating with the goal of meeting multiple, often conflicting, missions, in a demanding, constantly changing environment [1–4]. Many consider healthcare to be a service industry. However, comparisons cannot be made between other service-based industries such as utility providers (water or electricity), as these industries are not required to operate in a system with conflicting demands. Their goal is singular in that they strive to provide their particular service to their customers. Hospitals, on the other hand, are accountable to multiple stakeholder groups, including physicians, nurses, allied health professionals, government bodies, community partners, insurers, and, most importantly, patients [1]. Like schools, or first-response providers (fire, police, or ambulance services for example), hospitals operate in complex systems where financial health is as much a priority as high quality care provision, service excellence, and employee development. The inherent complexity of the hospital system means that while lessons can be learned from other industries, comparisons between the two cannot easily be made [1, 4]. As an illustration, while a power utility provider is unable to anticipate profound temperature changes and the necessity for more energy production to compensate for additional air conditioning in the summer or heat in the winter, healthcare cannot anticipate fluctuations in disease prevalence (influenza outbreaks, for example) or rapid changes in medical practice. These factors are beyond the control of the utility company and the healthcare provider, but cannot be equated, as advances in healthcare, while providing benefit, may also lead to significant and unexpected cost, whereas there have been hot and cold snaps in the past that the utility provider can look to for guidance. The utility company can use past data to predict what might be needed, but hospitals need a broader and more innovative outlook to succeed, requiring visionary leaders and staff, a culture that supports the vision, and systems that provide tools and measures that make achieving the vision a reality.

R. Stuhler (✉)
The Hospital for Sick Children (SickKids),
Toronto, ON, Canada

The Institute for Health Policy, Management,
and Evaluation (IHPME), University of Toronto,
Toronto, ON, Canada
e-mail: rivanna.stuhler@sickkids.ca

M. A. Koyle
The Hospital for Sick Children (SickKids),
Toronto, ON, Canada

The Institute for Health Policy, Management,
and Evaluation (IHPME), University of Toronto,
Toronto, ON, Canada

Department of Surgery, University of Toronto School
of Medicine, Toronto, ON, Canada
e-mail: martin.koyle@sickkids.ca

© Springer Nature Switzerland AG 2019
D. Burke et al. (eds.), *Hospital Transformation*, https://doi.org/10.1007/978-3-030-15448-6_6

In order to meet the unique challenges the health care system faces, those within the system must be aware of factors that improve, or worsen, performance and provision of care, so as to mitigate circumstances that can lead to failure in hospitals, of which there are many. Ideally, these should be identified early—by front-line staff, middle management, or those on the senior executive level—in order to allow for change, improvement, and ideally, success. This chapter will examine some of these factors, particularly those within the control and scope of managers and leaders at all levels throughout the organization. It is equally important for a manager who oversees one or two individuals, or the CEO of the hospital, who is responsible for thousands of people, to be aware of, and comfortable with, the following factors, as ignorance of these factors can lead to poor performance and ultimately, failure [5]. These factors are leadership, culture, vision, information gathering and management systems, and planning processes.

Leadership

A strong leader is the key to any successful organization. Traits of good leaders have been widely studied and reported [2, 6–10]. Mannion, Davies, and Marshall (2005) suggest a collection of characteristics they regard as key in a strong leader, including being visible, approachable, accountable, and promoting a "can-do" culture in which employees at all levels are encouraged to play a part in changing and improving the organization. Firth-Cozens and Mowbray (2001) further characterize good leaders as intelligent, sociable, determined, and assertive. Leaders should demonstrate integrity, and while ideally being confident, should also be humble enough to recognize and learn from mistakes (their own, or those of their staff or organization) [7, 9, 11]. They are receptive and responsive to problems within the organization, and are openly appreciative of their employee base, helping develop staff potential with the ultimate goal of aligning their individual priorities with that of the organization [8]. Strong leaders articulate a clear and consistent message

about the vision, mission (or missions, plural, given the nature of the hospital environment), and values of the organization, and understand the benefits of using multiple channels of communication to disseminate this message [1, 6, 12]. While they may be committed to ensuring that the overall vision and likely multiple missions of the hospital are met, good leaders also have an in-depth understanding of the challenges in meeting these goals from the perspective of those on the front-line. This allows them to foster the creation of realistic plans for improvement, as well as buy-in for these plans from their staff [11, 13]. The best leaders, while supportive of their staff, are also never comfortable with the status quo, always looking to improve [8]. They are passionate about quality improvement and patient safety, and make this subject a true priority, rather than just word speak, at all levels within the organization. By doing this, they encourage all staff, from the board of directors down to those on the front-lines, to be involved in well thought out and cleverly executed improvement initiatives [6, 7, 10, 13, 14]. This focus on improvement is vitally important given the ever-changing nature of healthcare, and the constant pressure to perform clinically and financially, both from internal and external stakeholders. An emphasis on safety ideally leads to a culture of safety, critical in high reliability organizations (HROs) such as those within the aviation and train transportation industries [15, 16]. Healthcare organizations aspire to be like HROs, or indeed, become HROs, where error is the exception rather than the rule, constant scrutiny and questioning at all levels leads to sustained improvement, and where accountability exists on all levels [16, 17]. Strong leaders who exhibit those skills as outlined above, and believe in the ethos of the HRO tend to lead hospitals which are higher performing organizations. Their approach ensures that the hospital is set up to succeed as the objectives of the institution are clearly stated, and plans to meet those objectives reasonable and realistic based on the needs of the organization.

Conversely, underperforming, or failing, hospitals, are often defined by a lack of innovative, visionary leaders. Keroak et al (2007) looked at leadership characteristics associated with high- and low-performing hospitals. Leaders at the top-performing institutions exhibited most, if not all, of those qualities outlined above. The traits of leaders in lower-performing hospitals were similar to those discussed by Mannion, Davies, and Marshall (2005), most specifically being perceived as remote or distant, disinterested, and intimidating. These leaders did not make themselves visible or approachable, and staff did not feel them to be trustworthy or exhibit a high degree of integrity. In these hospitals, leadership was not receptive to input from staff, and those who challenged the status quo were perceived as threats and "troublemakers," and sometimes removed from their posts. Relationships between internal departments, and with external partners were often antagonistic, with conflicting priorities fighting for recognition, instead of an alignment of multiple priorities under the same overarching organizational umbrella noted in higher-performing hospitals helmed by strong leaders [1, 6, 10, 12, 13]. Weaker leaders such as these tend to be more autocratic in style, resulting in organizations that do not welcome collaborative change and make decisions based on individual priorities, rather than those of the hospital at large [5, 10, 13]. There is less clarity at the leadership level as to the vision and mission(s) of the hospital, and quality improvement (QI) is a more abstract concept, unconnected to the daily operation of the hospital [10], unlike in high-performing centres where QI is integrated into every aspect of the organization. Because these lower performing hospitals operate within a culture of blame, error is more likely to occur, and lessons are not always learned from mistakes. Again, the example of the HRO and the radical improvements in safety that came about with the institution of checklists, other similar tools, and a shift towards an open and honest environment is relevant [15, 16]. Hospitals run by poor leaders are more likely to be those where error is a constant, and where propagation of an environment where failure is more likely to occur is the daily reality.

In order to avoid failure, leaders and managers at every level must be aware of those characteristics exhibited by themselves, their colleagues, and their organizations, that lead to poor collaboration and communication, and ultimately result in suboptimal performance and failure. Leaders who are not self-reflective, who do not benchmark against the highest performing organizations, and who reject feedback and data that indicate a less than optimal performance open themselves up to failure. In contrast, those who recognize gaps and deficiencies and work to create a culture of constant improvement with a collective approach to enhancing care are more likely to see improvements in performance with the added benefit of improved overall culture, another factor that can lead to failure in hospitals.

Culture

The culture of a hospital is integral to the way in which the organization works. The type of culture, and the qualities prioritized within it contribute to how well an organization performs. Cultures are unique to an organization, each with its own distinctive flavour and qualities. However, a high performing organization is more likely to have a strong culture, one that encompasses the general qualities of what is seen as a good and productive culture, in addition to those traits distinct to the organization. Strong leaders tend to foster strong cultures, as their commitment towards corporate clarity, all-staff involvement, and a positive, "can-do" working environment encourages a philosophy of collaboration, innovation, creativity, and accountability [6, 17]. Staff members who feel listened to, appreciated, and valued are more likely to perform well, as opposed to those who feel they work in a culture of blame, are overworked and underappreciated, and are apprehensive to speak up when issues arise due to a fear of punitive measures being taken against them [6, 8, 10, 15]. The environment that the latter group work in breeds cynicism, distrust, skepticism, a marked decrease in perceived work-life quality, and a high tendency towards poor practice, as challenge, dissent, and an openness to change are taboo within the culture [10, 12, 14, 18, 19]. Within these hospitals may exist a strongly retained culture of hierarchy with strict expectations of loyalty to the senior executive from management at all levels [2]. In organizations like this, leaders often place priority on projects close to their own self-interests rather than looking at the broader needs of the organization and prioritizing accordingly [13]. Employees therefore feel disempowered to create change, collaborate, innovate, or report errors, and may indeed work to a lesser standard as a result of overwork, demotivation, and lack of appreciation, potentially leading to institutional failures [2, 10, 15, 17, 18]. One key element of a good culture that appears to be lacking in these more toxic cultures is a commitment to organizational accountability, often from the top down.

Accountability is a key component of a healthy culture. Maintaining accountability is important on many levels, relating to both staff, and the organization itself. Organizational accountability fosters an environment in which staff know that blame will not be placed on them for the failings of the institution [15]. This engenders personal accountability within the organization, leading to a culture of safety over blame [15, 17], or what is commonly referred to as a "just culture." A just culture is one in which there is a balance between personal and organizational accountability [15, 20]. There is a focus on reporting of errors in order to allow for reflection and improvement, as opposed to placing of blame. In this way, just cultures are also learning cultures, those where safety incidents, preventable or otherwise, are considered opportunities for improvement [15, 20]. Just cultures prioritize safety, and provide cultural infrastructures that encourage communication, questioning, collaboration, and open and honest reporting [15, 20]. Within a just culture, staff ultimately become more comfortable reporting errors or asking for help, as they know the organization supports them in their efforts to improve [10, 15, 17].

Cultures that encourage and celebrate improvements of all sizes and on all levels create a willingness amongst staff to be accountable for their own actions as they know their work is appreciated. When leaders are openly accountable, and lead by example, staff may be more willing to do the same [10]. Accountability on all levels fosters a collective culture that allows for the creation of a strong and potentially symbiotic relationship with internal and external stakeholders, strengthening the links between hospitals and their community providers, as well as enhancing the local health economy [6]. Those working internally and externally know that they are respected and valued, and so work more positively to meet the collective goals of the organization. Thus a just culture is the ideal, but not always the reality, as shifts away from more closed and rigidly hierarchical cultures towards those that are open, honest, and collaborative take a very long time, and a sustained and concerted effort.

Of course not all hospitals have purely "good" or "bad" cultures. Most organizations have leanings towards one, but exhibit elements of the other. In order to recognize and minimize failure, the type of culture prevalent in an organization must be recognized by management at all levels. Data from employee satisfaction surveys and internal or external reviews must be taken seriously, and addressed in a timely manner. Suboptimal results cannot be ignored, and should be addressed in a manner that fosters real change, both structural and cultural. The best organizations will use their setbacks as change and growth opportunities, thus improving the culture [11, 13]. Results highlighting the successes of an organization should not be ignored either, as the continuation of these successes and maintenance of a good and just culture requires ongoing work. To do this requires a level of managerial and organizational humility, a strong institutional vision to aspire to, and a willingness to recognize that there are flaws within the structure and culture of the organization that could be improved upon. Failure to recognize this propagates a toxic culture that leads to poor practice and performance, attrition, and ultimately, a failing hospital.

Vision

In order for strong leaders to communicate a clear message about the vision and mission(s) of the organization to staff, a hospital must first ensure that a clear, overarching vision is in place. Hospitals, as complex organisms, generally have multiple missions under one vision [1–4]. There must be balance amongst the various mission statements in order to fully meet the vision, as this encourages collaboration amongst disparate stakeholder groups, both internal and external, and attempts to avoid competition between these stakeholders. Fostering collaboration over competition inspires stakeholders to embrace the organizational vision, and align their own individual priorities with those of the hospital [10]. A cohesive set of priorities organization-wide, supported by employees at every level, strengthens not only the culture of the hospital, but enhances the commitment of the entire organization to meeting the vision. Again, this brings into focus the need for an effective leader, a positive culture, and a clear organizational vision that staff and management feel aligned to. But vision is not only important at the executive level. West and Lyubovnikova (2013) discuss the importance of a vision at every level in the hospital, even for teams on the front lines, as calling a group a "team" does not automatically denote successful teamwork. Teams operate best when they have a vision in place, as well as clarity regarding the goals and mission of the team, responsibilities of the team members, and how the team should operate in order to succeed [2]. Ideally, to promote excellent service provision and achieve a high level of performance, the team's vision would be in line with the organization's vision and mission, and reflect the values of the hospital's culture. This allows for change that matches the goals of the organization, ultimately strengthening the team and the hospital as a whole [14].

A strong, well-thought out, and widely supported vision decreases the likelihood of large-scale failure, so long as consideration has been given to potential weaknesses that threaten the success of the vision [9]. Anyone can write what sounds to be a strong, viable vision, but in healthcare, with so many competing factors, strong leadership and a significant amount of thoughtfulness is required to achieve success. When leaders become complacent with the vision, and stop constantly reviewing it, the emphasis on continual improvement and system enhancement drops off, leading to a higher likelihood of poor performance and potential failure. Diligent leaders who relentlessly revisit the vision of their institution are more likely to see where it is succeeding, failing, and where optimization needs to occur to engender success.

Information Gathering and Management Systems

In order to create effective change and perform at the highest possible level, hospitals need to know what and how to change. This requires effective information systems and tools that allow providers to do their work, as well as collecting information that can be used by the hospital to create plans for improvement. Kutyla, Meyer, and Silow-Carroll (2004) stress the importance of investing in information technologies (IT) and tools that meet the needs of both providers and hospital administrators. This requires consultation with, and buy-in from, staff at all levels. Staff on every level should have input as to which tools are needed to enhance their day-to-day work, and the work of the hospital as a whole, as choosing the wrong system can have disastrous effects for an organization, as noted by Golden (2006). Many organizations feel that "more is better," but this is not always the case. More tools do not necessarily mean better, more efficient work-flows, and more useful information gathering. Indeed, having too many tools available may mean that some are used, and others abandoned. In this instance, there is the chance that the wrong tools are used, and some excellent options discarded, potentially to the detriment of patients, staff, and the organization as a whole. As such, staff need to be involved in every step involved in choosing data systems and tools, and deciding which metrics to prioritize to enhance the efficacy and impact of these systems [6]. In terms of information gathering and management systems, the biggest way a hospital could fail is by spending millions of dollars or pounds on a system and set of tools that collect the wrong information, or information that is auxiliary to the needs of the hospital, and is despised by the employee base. Thus the importance of careful vetting of any system and heavy involvement from staff at all levels cannot be underscored.

Let us assume that a hospital has succeeded in choosing and implementing an IT system that works well for staff and management. In order to ensure continued success, the hospital must focus on ongoing measurement and data analysis to allow for continuous improvement initiatives and effective streamlining of services [13]. But first they must determine what those measures are. Keroak et al (2007) discuss the importance of using tools effectively in order to determine a set of metrics that can be used objectively across an entire organization to make clear those initiatives which would be most impactful to the organization and ideally achieve higher performance. Choosing the right tools keeps organizations on their toes, and constantly evolving. Reason (2000) notes that the right tools remind organizations not to become too comfortable with the status quo by reinforcing that constant improvement is the goal. The right system and tools are as vital to a hospital's success as a strong leader, positive culture and clear vision are, as they help plot the future direction of the organization, ideally setting it up to succeed.

Planning Processes

Hospitals are constantly having to change the way in which they work. However, success is only achieved when change and improvement initiatives are carefully thought out, planned, and executed. One of the most common ways in which hospitals fail is by creating initiatives without first considering the change needs of the organization [21, 22]. The first potential failure opportunity for an organization is to propose a change that does not match the needs of the hospital or local health economy, and so is perceived by those within the system to be a waste of time and money [3]. If this is the perception, there will be no buy-in from staff, and less motivation to support or accept the change. Completing a needs assessment and involving stakeholders in

the planning process can mitigate potential failure, and quash plans destined to be ineffective. In the case where a change has been deemed necessary, leadership can foster support and maximize the proposed change's chance of success by making a strong case for the initiative, allowing staff to ask questions about the plan, and make suggestions that might improve the process [12, 13]. Staff may be able to provide suggestions that allow planned interventions to be effective on multiple levels, ultimately benefitting the hospital. Regardless of the strength of a proposed initiative, it is likely to fail without adequate increases in capacity, resources, infrastructure, and equipment to support the change [5, 13]. Leaders who do not consider the potential weaknesses of a proposed plan, and how it will affect those required to carry out and follow the plan are more likely to fail, as staff will perceive their commitment to the project as less than optimal, and will be less motivated to support the intervention when implemented. Completing a pre-mortem and "planning to fail" by considering all potential weaknesses during the planning process can help leaders hone a plan and increase its chance of success [9, 23]. Failed projects cost organizations time and money, and can erode employee trust and commitment. This can affect the culture of an organization, and its overall performance as. Careful consideration of all aspects of a change—the cost, the required resources, and the potential impacts, both positive and negative, can help an organization avoid complete failure of the planned intervention.

Conclusion

It is easiest to understand why hospitals fail if we have a good understanding of the factors that allow institutions to succeed. By acknowledging and understanding those factors that help hospitals excel, we can more easily pinpoint the things that are missing in hospitals that are underperforming, or failing. In order to see early those things leading their hospitals towards failure, it is essential that leaders and managers have a broad understanding of the unique issues faced by hospitals, and a grasp of those factors that contribute to excellence, or, on the other side of the spectrum, suboptimal performance, and ultimately, failure.

References

1. Golden B. Transforming healthcare organizations. Healthc Q. 2006;10:10–9.
2. West MA, Lyubovnikova L. Illusions of team working in health care. J Health Organ Manag. 2013;27(1):134–42.
3. Taylor MJ, McNicholas C, Nicolay C, Darzi A, Bell D, Reed JE. Systematic review of the application of the plan-do-study-act method to improve quality in healthcare. BMJ Qual Saf. 2014;23:290–8.
4. Edmonstone J. Organisational learning. In: Godbole P, Burke D, Aylott J, editors. Why hospitals fail: between theory and practice. Cham: Springer; 2017. p. 129–35.
5. Kutyla T, Meyer J, Silow-Carroll S. Hospital quality: ingredients for success – overview and lessons learned. Commonwealth Fund. 2004. http://www.commonwealthfund.org/publications/fund-reports/2004/jul/hospital-quality-ingredients-success-overview-and-lessons. Accessed 20 July 2018.
6. Mannion R, Davies HTO, Marshall MN. Cultural characteristics of "high" and "low" performing hospitals. J Health Organ Manag. 2005;19(6):431–9.
7. Firth-Cozens J, Mowbray D. Leadership and the quality of care. Qual Health Care. 2001;10(Suppl 2):ii3–7.
8. Taylor N, Clay-Williams R, Hogden E, Braithwaite J, Groene O. High performing hospitals: a qualitative review of associated factors and practical strategies for improvement. BMC Health Serv Res. 2015;15:244–64.
9. Mills JKA, McKimm J. Pre-empting project failure by using a pre-mortem. Br J Hosp Med. 2005;78(10):584–5.
10. Keroak MA, Youngberg BJ, Cerese JL, Krsek C, Prellwitz LW, Trevelyan EW. Organizational factors associated with high performance in quality and safety in academic medical centers. Acad Med. 2007;82:1178–86.
11. Reason J. Human error: models and management. BMJ. 2000;320:768–70.
12. Bell R, Golden B, Lee L. Transforming healthcare organizations – looking back to see the future. Healthc Q. 2006;10:84–7.
13. Longenecker PD, Longenecker CO. Why hospital improvement efforts fail: a view from the front line. J Healthc Manag. 2014;59(2):147–57.
14. Puoane T, Cuming K, Sanders S, Ashworth A. Why do some hospitals achieve better care of severely malnourished children than others? Five-year follow-up of rural hospitals in Eastern Cape, South Africa. Health Policy Plan. 2008;23(6):428–37.
15. Boysen PG II. Just culture: a foundation for balanced accountability and patient safety. Ochsner J. 2013;13(3):400–6.
16. Wachter RM, Gupta K. Creating a culture of safety. In: Wachter RM, Gupta K, editors. Understanding patient safety. 3rd ed. New York: McGraw-Hill Education; 2018. p. 281–306.
17. Rodziewicz TL, Hipskind JE. Medical error prevention. StatPearls [Internet]. Treasure Island: StatPearls Publishing; 2018. https://www.ncbi.nlm.nih.gov/books/NBK499956/. Accessed 20 July 2018.
18. Cornish J, Jones A. Factors affecting compliance with moving and handling policy: student nurses' views and experiences. Nurse Educ Pract. 2010;10(2):96–100.
19. Wachter RM, Gupta K. Workforce issues. In: Wachter RM, Gupta K, editors. Understanding patient safety. 3rd ed. New York: McGraw-Hill Education; 2018. p. 307–30.
20. Patient Safety Culture. Canadian Patient Safety Institute. 2018. http://www.patientsafetyinstitute.ca/en/toolsResources/PatientSafetyIncidentManagementToolkit/PatientSafetyManagement/pages/patient-safety-culture.aspx. Accessed 20 Aug 2018.
21. Brand CA, Barker AL, Morello RT, Vitale MR, Evans SM, Scott IA, Stoelwinder JU, Cameron PA. A review of hospital characteristics associated with improved performance. Int J Qual Health Care. 2012;24(5):483–94.
22. McMillan K. Politics of change: the discourses that inform organizational change and their capacity to silence. Nurs Inq. 2016;23(3):223–31.
23. Carayon P, Xie A, Kianfar S. Human factors and ergonomics as a patient safety practice. BMJ Qual Saf. 2014;23:196–205.

The Illness of the Health Care Systems

Jaime Llambías-Wolff

Introduction

The fiscal crisis of the state paired with current demographic and epidemiological transitions are critically challenging health care systems. They appear to be unsustainable in the face of the increasing cost of care and related expenses, the significant financial impact of chronic disease, the over-consumption of pharmaceuticals, unaffordable technologies [1–4] and an increasing demand for quality and quantity of health care. This global crisis—affecting both the private and the public health care systems [5–12]—has been fully documented for no less than three decades. Due to the limitations of this curative ideology, [13–16] neither the emergence of a sophisticated private medical sector nor the deteriorating public health care system can respond effectively to these critical challenges as they both do not address or challenge the hegemony of the paradigm itself.

Though different schools of thought have generated a noteworthy body of literature, relatively little analysis has attempted to bridge these critiques. As there have been a number of alternative paradigms put forth [7, 17–20], it is perhaps worth examining why suggested change within the health field has been so slow.

The objective of this chapter is to explore contemporary contentious issues within the health field in hopes of opening and facilitating the debate for alternative responses. For the purpose of a more comprehensive future analysis, these global critical issues have been organized into four categories: (1) Epistemological Issues; (2) Science and Knowledge; (3) Power Relations and the Political Economy and (4) Alternative Approaches and Practical Implications.

Epistemological Issues

In relation to epistemology, several critical contentious issues appear to be recurrent in the contemporary debate. Primarily, the limitations of the biomedical model appear to be one of the main obstacles for overcoming the health crisis itself [14, 21, 22]. In re-discovering and re-visiting the thoughts, views and learning experiences of the seventeenth and nineteenth centuries, there is a renewed emphasis on focusing upon social determinants, an integrated approach, the valuable input of subjective factors, the role of society and the importance of politics, economics and philosophy in the health field.

It appears that long after the World Health Organization's (WHO) declaration that health is not merely the absence of disease, modern medicine is still focused upon illness and infection rather than structurally-based social issues surrounding health [23]. Despite this biomedical bias, demographic

J. Llambías-Wolff (✉)
York University, Toronto, ON, Canada
e-mail: jlwolff@yorku.ca

and epidemiological transitions—along with rising costs of medical technologies, fiscal crises of the welfare states, as well as the business approach of the emerging medical-industrial-service sector—are forcing theorists to deconstruct the hegemonic notion of the health-disease equation. As a result, pluralist and transdisciplinary ideologies are in increased demand due to the overarching need for a paradigm shift in health.

It is through these failures of the biomedical ideology that a stigma has begun to develop against modern, biomedical, or pharmaceutically based treatments [24]. However, despite this growing stigma and its related augmented interest in alternative health perspectives, there is still a need for biomedical treatments with respect to the biological relationship to pathogens within the human body. Nevertheless, the impacts of biomedicine's historical roots are significant and undeniable. With ties deeply rooted within concepts of dualism, reductionism as well as the popularized "mechanical analogy" [25], biomedical demand is placing increased pressure on the allocation and availability of medical resources. These resources—already in short supply—are found to be more tightly stretched than in previous years, in particular due to the emergence of a needier ageing population who tend to experience higher rates of chronic disease and discomfort.

Infectious diseases on the other hand are becoming less of a focus for researchers compared to previous years and instead are of more casual interest. This shift in research priority is the result of an increased occurrence of antibiotic resistance [26], the emergence and re-emergence of contagious diseases, tobacco use, sedentary lifestyles, as well as malnutrition and obesity across an array of both developed and developing nations. Health crises such as these suggest a biomedical incapacity and/or incapability in the face of more structurally based health problems that do not necessarily have direct roots in the physical fundamentals of the biological onset of disease.

Due to the inability to effectively respond to such issues, emerging alternative paradigms are seen as a "movement of criticism against the dominant paradigm" [27] of biomedicine, suggesting the current "biomedical monolithic worldview" [28] ignores what lies between or beyond its borders [27]. Transitions toward alternative health care practices and reformed public health policy currently highlight the restrictions and "inadequacies" of biomedicine, rather than alter the foundational perspectives and understandings of health and illness. There is a need for health perspectives and health care itself to become "more sensitive, critical and responsive" [29] to the demands of one's physical, psychological and spiritual being. Such concepts of health and disease reflect how health ought to be cured and managed [30], yet there is currently not a strong unifying alternative perspective outside the domineering biomedical ideology.

Using satisfaction user as indicator of success or a need for change, the humanization of health care is thus possible and serves as an aid for reconstructing existing health care models [31]. It is this humanization process [32] that allows for a more subjective evaluation of health; widening the definition of success regardless of what respect the health care comes from. In transitioning away from a narrow science-based legitimacy, governments are also recognizing the significance of ethics and the "social dimension of health" [33–35].

In order to promote the potential for innovative views and changes, there is a need for a transdisciplinary "weltanschauung" (cosmovision). A pluralistic approach to a reconstructed health paradigm as opposed to a "hyperdiscipline" is crucial as it "proposes dialogue between the sciences, the arts, literature [and] human experience" [27]. First and foremost, issues of complexity, logic and numerous realities must be addressed [27] and not ignored. Such complexities pave the way for questions regarding how deeply entrenched the existing monolithic paradigm is to modern society as well as its potential for change.

Science and Knowledge

As Engel [21] expresses, there are a variety of limitations set out by the current scientific paradigm that allow for the development of refined health care models. It is through these developments in research, education and health care that the integration of alternative modalities, followed by public policy reform, has been emerging. According to Plack [36], the potential for a complete paradigm shift relies on research, as its fuelling mechanism. Plack [36] outlines how it is crucial to include the views of the researchers—public policy makers, government officials, and related industries—as well as those considered stakeholders or 'consumers' in today's health market economy as part of the decision-making process.

However, governments concerned with the production and efficiency of health care systems demand that alternative methods be evaluated for legitimacy. Often, this is accomplished objectively against scientific fact rather than a more subjective or inclusive evaluative method. Though current health research is expanding towards inter- and transdisciplinary approaches, this must occur within all facets of health to ensure a successful transition to invigorated approaches. Though objectivity is at the foundation of the development of science, we shall also integrate the subjectivity of alternative methods, thus offering wider standards of legitimacy as the basis upon which emerging paradigms can prosper.

Alternative health paradigms are also stunted by research capacity, as there are astounding differences in funding between biomedical versus public health research [37]. A double standard exists such that complementary and alternative medicine (CAM) must be "evidence-based" in order to merit research time and funding. If the acquisition and products of the research do not fit within biomedical frameworks, related concepts of medical pluralism remain "relatively ignored" [38]. Due to such narrow research perspectives and legitimacy issues, CAM is placed at a further disadvantage with respect to its development and integration. Therefore research circles should promote collective and innovative perspectives with respect to current health issues and their consequent solutions [39]. There is a need for a balanced incorporation of community-level action in tandem with properly aimed research to "inform evidence-based practice, social action, and effective policy change" [39].

Research programs are crucial in the development of a paradigm that encompasses the environment, biology, psychology as well as the social sciences [25]. At the same time by committing more research to alternative methods and emerging paradigms in health, we are also able to determine its limitations, restrictions, as well as directions for the future. Without a full understanding of the characteristics of this emerging paradigm, it is impossible to conclude that the development and incorporation of alternative methods would improve health care quality and be conducive to increased accessibility. Also, medical curricula that trains health professionals in biomedical and alternative methods, for example, has been effective in developing holistic health perspectives for practitioners and patients alike, suggesting a potential break through in future developments dedicated to improving the current health crises from the ground up.

Power Relations and the Political Economy

Power relations and the political economy of health have animated the intellectual debate for decades—many health issues themselves are contradictory. Although they are intertwined economically and politically, these issues relate to intangible, elusive and sometimes ethereal concepts. They can simultaneously be the object and the result of change, as well as the instrument of maintaining the status quo. Health changes need to be explained with reference to the economic conditions and various interests they sustain, where people are seen not as autonomous individuals, but as actors within specific social locations and relationships. In addition, the role of the State and the impact of economic activity cannot be viewed as an autonomous entity in relation to institutional and legal conceptual constraints. As social structure induces and influences human activity, human activity is in turn necessary for its reproduction.

When the concept of social welfare emerged globally in 1945, most developed capitalist countries adopted a doctrine sustaining the Beveridge Report in tandem with Keynesian economic policy. We should recall that Beveridge, while trying to cope with the circumstances of war, attempted to ease the prevalent social inequality through social security and other government subsidies. Moreover, the Keynesian theory proposed to mitigate the effects of economic depression by acting on demand through the State. The implementation and further development of both conceptualizations gave rise to what is known as the Welfare State. Both right and moderate left wing political parties carried out this policy, with its most ardent defenders being social democratic governments.

Today, neo-liberal reforms have changed the relationship between State and society [40]. International financial institutions have played—and continue to play—a significant role in the formation of social policy, particularly in areas of health and pension programs. Social security reforms have been promoted by World Bank loans whereby the market is responsible for providing health and pensions. By default, the State is responsible for the poor and with limited financial resources this can only mean incomplete access for health care [41]. According to Hart [42], there are a variety of issues on the rise with respect to the future directions for health and health care delivery that are currently at the mercy of industrialization and political action. Amongst these issues lies the public versus private debate, a struggle to determine optimal health production, which has been generously publicized by popular media in recent times. Whether by a lack of interest or the existence of alternate agendas, the demands and desires of the population as a whole are not being accommodated. Meanwhile, those who benefit most from the current health care system, social structure and economic system continue to do so.

Nevertheless, in the current context of the liberalization of a globalized economy and of fiscal inability to assume all costs of benefits, it is virtually impossible to imagine a return to the Welfare State, or to dramatically reverse the privatization processes. Also, it shall be recognized that the growing so-called "middle class" is often caught between a public sector—with enormous difficulties to satisfy their health care needs—and their own economic capacity to resort to private medicine. This demographic has benefited from extending private health insurances.

Despite the dominant approach, there has been a distinct change in health perspectives with regards to the use, promotion and integration of alternative health care services. Questions arise as to whether the changing views of health and illness can be attributed to the citizens who are currently using complimentary alternative practices. This population perhaps consists of the wealthier "upper class" that are most likely to afford these less popular and consequently generally more expensive treatments. However, this demographic is primarily made up of the less well-off in search of alternative healing modalities to avoid expensive treatment plans. There is potential that governments could also be promoting these changing perspectives of health and illness in an attempt to accommodate increased numeric and fiscal demand on the health care system and the burden on current services. Nevertheless, this transition towards a paradigm shift requires social empowerment and activism, inferring a population of politically involved citizens in association with governments that lobby for the needs of the population as an entire entity.

Alternatives, Approaches and Practical Implications

Through alternative and natural approaches to health, the limitations and counter productivity of modernization, urbanization and industrialization are forced under the spotlight. At times, these failures infer worsened health effects [24] as opposed to the improved health for which they are intended. Alternative health approaches (such as holistic worldview, cultural synergies, traditional practices, spirituals movements, re-inventing social health, natural approaches, herbalists, natural therapies, etc.) are responses to the health crisis and intend to explore a better understanding of health and health determinants and develop a solid and balance relationship between humans and their living physical and social environment. Some alternative theorists see health as a "patterned, emergent, unpredictable, unitary, intuitive and innovative view" where the human body is seen as a "dynamic field of energy" [30]. Others focus on the body's health-promoting relationship with nature and its reciprocal physical and psychological health benefits [43]. In recent times, the emergence of a more holistic worldview of health encompassing the environment, biology, psychology, social science and other aspects, has been suggested as a reasonable dialogue between the sciences, philosophy, the arts, literature, human experience, etc.

This converge has begun to emerge with forefronts in public health policy, patient advocacy, as well as the inclusion of complementary and alternative medicine (CAM) into the existing biomedical model. Although CAM is criticized for a lack of legitimate structure in theory and practice, the resurgence of alternative therapies—especially during an accelerated time of technological advancement—suggests biomedicine has very clear restrictions and 'inadequacies' [44]. As such, there is a growing popularity of integrative medicine within a variety of health care settings and progressive health policies [28]. As populations conceptualize health in different ways [23], there is a need to accommodate a variety of health realities within a new paradigm, parallel with the integrative skills of physicians in the changing global environment [45].

The population involvement and the practical implications within the emerging paradigm are also present in the field of health promotion, as this category of social communication is also instrumental for social development [46]. Though it has been criticized for representing an economically sound escape from tackling structural problems by placing onus upon individuals for their own health, health promotion has been a mechanism for presenting broader health concepts. Health promotion exists upon the assumption that governments are in charge of altering health perspectives and consequently, paradigms.

New health paradigms must be built upon strong foundations and call for a balanced incorporation of community-based feedback as well as social action, and effective policy change. Through these processes there stands an augmented obligation for a negotiated consensus among key stakeholders in order to identify and prioritize health targets within regional community programming frameworks [47].

Refreshingly, the new approaches do not merely focus on the managerial, funding or organizational aspects of health services. It is noteworthy that alternative health movements shed light upon the collective and more pluralistic perspectives of current health issues in adopting new ways of thinking.

Conclusion

The dominance of biomedicine is very apparent within current discussions regarding global health crises, creating much speculation for what must be done to yield improved health results in years to come. Facing resource shortages, rising health care costs, heated political climates as well as economic markets spinning seemingly out of control, the health of populations is at stake such that the effects of these factors are now potentially irreversible and unavoidable. In hopes of suggesting reformed and innovative views at improving and achieving health, new alternative paradigms emerge as answers that are only being partially explored. Due to the strict guidelines of biomedicine and scientific objectivity, these alternative methods face problems of legitimacy and stunted development through incomplete funding and research strategies, as well as a lack of political advocacy.

Though change in perspectives, validity of practice and political determination have begun, the ball is slow-rolling, in that focus still remains upon expensive medical technologies and treatments intended to cure illness and disease rather than the social determinants and an altered social structure. Health must be perceived as a humanistic product whereby the mechanisms to achieve it are socially specific and accommodating of one's mind, body, spirit, ethnicity, race, gender and social and economic circumstances. To accomplish this feat, inclusive and inter- and trans-disciplinary approaches must be adapted by emerging health paradigms and the consequent health care system, in hopes of meeting the surmounting health crises and providing sustainability in health for the future. Whether the industrialization and commodification of health is irreversible or not, we must make a valiant effort to understand and dissect the mechanisms and structures underpinning the current circumstance in order to move forward with new, innovative and revisited ideas.

References

1. Carlson RJ. Breakthroughs in Biomedical Technology. In: Schwartz H, Karl C, editors. Dominant issues in medical sociology. Don Mills: Addison-Wesley; 1978.
2. Cassels A. Health sector reform: key issues in less developed countries, document WHO/SPS/NHP/95.4. Geneva: World Health Organization; 1995.
3. Fox N. Medical technology: a postmodern view. In: Postmodernism, sociology and health. Toronto: University of Toronto Press; 1994.
4. Kaufman S. Medicines' means and ends, 1970s-1990s: technological superiority, moral confusion. In: Sharon, R. Kaufman, The healer's tale. Wisconsin: The University of Wisconsin Press; 1993.
5. Crawford R. C'est de ta faute: l'Idéologie de la culpabilisation de la victime et ses applications dans les politiques de santé. In Bozzini L, et al., Médecine et Société-les Années 80. Québec: Éditions Coopératives Albert Saint-Martin; 1981.
6. Heubner A. The Non-Win War on Cancer East-West: The Journal of Natural Health and Living. en: Daniel E, editor. Taking Sides. The Dushkin Publishing Group; 1993.
7. Illich I. Némesis Médicale: l'expropriation de la Santé, Paris, Éd. Seuil. 1975.
8. McKeown T. Les déterminants de l'état de santé des populations depuis trois siècles: le comportement, l'environnement et la médecine. In: Bozzini, et al., op. cit. 1981.
9. Powles J. On the limitations of modern medicine. Sci Med Man. 1973;1(1):1–30.
10. Renaud M. Crise de la médecine et politiques de santé: leçons de l'histoire. In: Possibles, Vol. 2, No. 2, Montréal, Winter. 1977
11. Rossman M. The orthodox and unorthodox in health care. Soc Policy. 1975;6(1):28–30.
12. Zola I. Culte de la santé et méfaits de la médicalisation. In: Bozzini, et al., Médecine et Société: les Années 80, op. cit. 1981.
13. Bozzini L, Renaud M, Gaucher D, Llambías-Wolff J. Médicine et Société-les Années 80. Québec: Éditions Coopératives Albert Saint-Martin; 1981.
14. Capra F. The biomedical model. In: The turning point: science, society, and the rising culture. London: Fontanta; 1982.
15. Lupton D. The Lay Perspective on Illness and Disease. In: Medicine as culture: illness, disease and the body in western societies. London: Sage; 1994.
16. Turner A. Concepts of Disease and Sickness: Women's Complaints: Patriarchy and Illness. In: Medical power and social knowledge. London: Sage; 1987.
17. Gordon, J. Conversations: James Gordon, MD, connecting mind, body and beyond. In: Alternative therapies in health & medicine, March/April. 2006.
18. Gordon J. Asian spiritual traditions and their usefulness to practioners and patients facing life and death. J Altern Complement Med. 2002;8(5):603–8.
19. Le Fanu J. The rise and fall of modern medicine. New York: Carroll & Graf; 2000.
20. Schneirov M, Geczic JD. Alternative health: from livehood to politics. Albany: State University of New York; 2003.
21. Engel GL. The need for a new medical model: a challenge for biomedicine. In: Marks DF, editor. The health psychology reader. London: Sage; 1977. p. 50–65.
22. Wade D, Halligan P. Do biomedical models of illness make for good health care systems? Br Med J. 2004;329:1398–401.
23. Levin BW, Browner CH. The social production of health: critical contributions from evolutionary, biological, and cultural anthropology. Soc Sci Med. 2005;61(4):745–50.
24. Wayland C. The failure of pharmaceuticals and the power of plants: medicinal discourse as a critique of modernity in the Amazon. Soc Sci Med. 2004;58(12):2409–19.
25. Longino CF Jr. The limits of scientific medicine: paradigm strain and social policy. J Health Soc Policy. 1998;9(4):101–16.
26. Pfeiffer J, et al. What can critical medical anthropology contribute to global health? A health systems perspective. Med Anthropol Quart. 2008;22(4):410–5.
27. de Alvarenga AT, Sommerman A, Alvarez AMDS. International congresses on transdisciplinarity: reflections on emergences and convergences of ideas and ideals towards a new modern science. Saude Soc [online]. 2005;14(3):9–29.
28. Hollenberg D, Muzzin L. Health Sociol Rev. 2010;19(1):34–56.
29. Ayres JRCM. A hermeneutical concept of health. Physis [online]. 2007;17(1):43–62.
30. Newman MA. Health as expanding consciousness. 2nd ed. Sudbury: Jones & Bartlett; 2000. p. 3–13.

31. Costa GD, Da Cotta RMM, do Franceschini SCC, Rodrigo S, Andreia P, Cardoso P, da Silva Marques Ferreira M d L. Health evaluation: reflections on contemporary sanitary paradigms. Physis: Revista de Saude Coletiva. 2008;18(4):705–26.

32. Goldberg JD. Humanism or professionalism? the white coat ceremony and medical education. Acad Med. 2008;83(8):715–22.

33. Bolaria BS, Bolaria R. Personal and structural determinants of health and illness: lifestyles and life chances. In: Bolaria BS, Dickinson HD, editors. Health, ilness, and health care in Canada. Nelson: Thomson Learning; 2002. p. 445–59.

34. Marmot M. Social determinants of health inequalities. Lancet. 2005;365(9464):1099.

35. Raphael D. Social determinants of health: present status, unanswered questions, and future directions. Int J Health Serv. 2006;36(4):651–67.

36. Plack MM. Human nature and research paradigms: theory meets physical therapy practice. Qual Rep. 2005;10(2):223–45.

37. McCarthy M. Innovation. Eur J Soc Sci Res. 2010;23(1):69–77.

38. Kaptchuk TJ, Miller FG. Viewpoint: what is the best and most ethical model for the relationship between mainstream and alternative medicine: opposition, integration, or pluralism? Acad Med. 2005;80(3):286–90.

39. Dankwa-Mullan I, et al. Moving toward paradigm-shifting research in health disparities through translation, transformational, and trans-disciplinary approaches. Am J Public Health. 2010;100(S1):S19–24.

40. Fleury S. Reshaping Health Care in Latin America: toward Fairness? In: Fleury S, Belmartino S, Baris E, editors. Reshaping Health Care in Latin America, Chap. 9. IDRC; 2000.

41. Berlinguer G. Globalization and global health. Int J Health Serv. 1999;29(3):579–95.

42. Hart TJ. Health care or health trade? A historic moment of choice. Int J Health Serv. 2004;34(2):245–54. Retrieved from MEDLINE database.

43. Hansen-Ketchum P, Marck P, Reutter L. Engaging with nature to promote health: new directions for nursing research. J Adv Nurs. 2009;65(7):1527–38.. Retrieved from EBSCOhost

44. Shupe A, Hadden JK. Spiritual healing and the medical model. North Central Sociological Association; 1998.

45. Hsiao AF, Ryan GW, Hays RD, Coulter ID, Andersen RM, Wenger NS. Variations in provider conceptions of integrative medicine. Soc Sci Med. 2006;62(12):2973–87.

46. Gumucio-Dargon A. "When the doctor does not know," critical remarks on health promotion, communication and participation. Estudios sobre las culturas contemporáneas. 2010;16(31):67–93.

47. Scheid TL, Joyner DR, Plescia MG, Blasky K. Steps to a negotiated consensus: a framework for developing community health initiatives. Res Sociol Health Care. 2006;24:235–57.

The Political Economy of Health Reforms in Chile: A Case Study of the Privatization Process

Jaime Llambías-Wolff

Introduction

Health issues are contradictory. Although they are intertwined economically and politically, they relate to intangible, elusive and sometimes ethereal concepts. They can simultaneously be the object and the result of change, and the instrument of status-quo. Health reforms need to be explained with reference to the economic conditions and the various interests they sustain, where people are seen not as autonomous individuals but as actors within specific social locations and relationships. Therefore, the question: "who benefits?" is essential to uncover the process of health reforms.

An analysis of the way power is employed to influence policies, reforms and legislation remains sometimes neglected or underestimated. How has Chilean socio-economic and political development influenced and shaped the different health models and reforms? How was hegemony built into the process of implementing health reforms? What were the ideological, economic and socio-political factors behind these health reforms?

The context of health reforms in Latin America and in Chile was more the articulation of conflicting interests in the political arena, mediated by the political strength and mobilization capacity of

the political actors and the organized civil society, as well as the armed forces. Governments have bargained with labor factions, urban workers, employees, the police and the armed forces separately, ultimately resulting in a very heterogeneous structure, where the rights and benefits of these factions have come to depend on the negotiation power of the stakeholders Murdock [1] and [2].

This chapter discusses the evolution of the Chilean health care system along with the result of negotiations that transpired between a web of economic, political and cultural forces during the following time periods where crucial health reforms were implemented.

Theoretical Concerns

Changes to the health care system must be considered in light of the broader social, economic and political factors. According to Frenk, a Health System can be understood as *"a set of relationships among major groups of actors: the health care providers, the population, the State as a collective mediator, the organizations that generate resources, and the other sectors that produce services with health effects"* [3, p. 19]. From a comparative perspective all countries have similar concerns, but the economic, political, ideological and epidemiological reasons behind them differ. Social reforms have also an ambiguous character. In the process of deepening social reforms we are

J. Llambías-Wolff (✉)
York University, Toronto, ON, Canada
e-mail: jlwolff@yorku.ca

© Springer Nature Switzerland AG 2019
D. Burke et al. (eds.), *Hospital Transformation*, https://doi.org/10.1007/978-3-030-15448-6_8

confronted with a plurality of objectives that correspond to different interests. This process has also a paradoxical, but probably necessary dialectical nature: it facilitates equity, promotes protection and democratizes society, while also legitimizing the State and a system of power that has created its own inequality and lack of protection.

As indicated by Fitzpatrick in relation to the development of the Welfare State: *"since a welfare democracy would require a more egalitarian distribution of power and resources as exists at present, we need an account of those from whom power and resources would need to be redistributed"* [4, p. 12]. The Welfare State has improved income distribution, but has also influenced and affected the accumulation of capital. On the other hand, it has also induced changes in labour productivity, but deepened as well many of the values and rights that workers have acquired over time.

In addition, the role of the State and the impact of economic activity cannot be viewed as an autonomous entity in relation to institutional and legal conceptual constraints. Social structures induce and influence social and human activity, but social activity is also necessary for the reproduction of the social structure. Therefore, within a larger political context the need is to secure conditions for this reproduction and the constructing of hegemony. Poulantzas argues that classes and social groups have many different determinations, which consequently require a negotiation of interests through a block that *"constitutes a contradictory unity of politically dominant classes and fractions, under the protection of the hegemonic fraction"* [5, p. 239].

For Gramsci, who anticipated much of the work done by the structuralists, neo-marxist, structural-marxists like Althusser [6] and later by poststructuralists and post-modernists: *"The hegemonic process is then defined not simply on the basis of the relations between groups, but on the basis of the relations between groups and structures"* [7, p. 178]. By conceptualizing that the super-structure may have autonomy with respect to the infrastructure, and bearing in mind that orthodox historical materialism did not consider this in the same terms, the Gramscian interpretation left the door open to the possibility of

a non-mechanistic interpretation of the processes of creating law and of the confrontation of interests, negotiation and the dynamic role of ideology. Neo-Gramscian analysis views hegemony as a terrain of struggle where social prevalent ideas must be constantly articulated and rearticulated at the various levels of the social structure Gill [8], Rupert [9] and Augelli and Murphy [10]. The concept of hegemony is essentially a concept that expresses a form of domination, which is exercised in different ways and also originates in lawful ways, but it is invariably linked to power relations and the power structure in a society. For this reason, it is important to examine how the State acts and reacts in this process, where hegemony is exercised.

The role of the State is critical, since it "acts as strategic terrain for the implementation of hegemonic projects" and it is the site of major struggles as well as negotiations, compromises, consent, articulations, inclusions and exclusions [11, p. 183]. This is similarly noted by Barton when he states that, *"theories of social contract, of hegemony and of class struggle all refer to these changing social relations and how the State is then co-opted by different social groups for different ends"* [12, p. 361].

Conflict among stakeholders to intervene in the process of health policies and the delivery of health care services is a constant struggle. Influence and capability of mobilizing interest groups on health reforms have historically been important in several Latin American countries. This is particularly interesting, since Health Systems in Latin America are characterized as being fragmented systems [13, p. 170; 14, pp. 162–116]. It is difficult to classify them as purely public or private, due to the complex arrangements and negotiations that are the result of political choices Heidenheimer et al. [15]. Systems of social protection, differing in each country, have been formed through diverse historical development. These social protection systems are developed through a combination of economic, political and cultural forces. These forces, along with unique sets of social values shared by the population, form a complex web of institutions "responsible for financing, organizing and providing social service delivery", which define "who is entitled to benefits and services" [16, p. 1].

Countries in Latin America were left with a very stratified health care system; workers in the formal labor market were entitled to social security benefits, while the rest of the population received services provided by the State, consequently creating differences and inequities amongst sectors. Latin America has developed its own system of social protection originating in profound economic, political, and cultural changes that accompanied the process of industrialization and urbanization. The role of the State became more interventionist in order to ensure emerging social rights [16, p. 1]. Also, as earlier discussed, the system was also determined by the dynamics of a power struggle between the important classes and social actors, and the ability to mobilize their goals and forge alliances to create temporary social consensus [16, 17, pp. 2014–2015].

Consequently, it is the implementation of a policy originating from above (the State) that generated a period of unprecedented economic growth, ensuring a standard of living, providing employment and basic social services (health, education, retirement), for the people of the countries that adopted such a pathway. For Fleury, *The concept of social protection in Latin America rested on social and institutional mechanisms of differentiation. Nevertheless, this political give-and take constituted the first instance in which the demands of the working class were considered in the political arena and incorporated in the government agenda"* (…) *Social protection was rooted in a political system wherein the State played a key role in the industrialization process by combining industrial protectionism with a controlled political incorporation of urban workers' demands"* [16, pp. 2–3].

The legitimacy of the State was built under a corporatist approach, following the European model. In England and Wales the Health System was built with an active participation of the working class, creating a hierarchical system with the provision of services according to levels of care. The consolidation of a national Health System was achieved thanks to several political contexts

and of a negotiation process between actors and interests at play [18, p. 75]. It is particularly interesting to note that the active participation of interest groups—in their various expressions—in national health reforms, began at the opening of the twentieth century, before the Welfare State.

When the concept of social welfare emerged in the world in the 1945s, most developed capitalist countries adopted the doctrine sustaining the Beveridge Report along with Keynesian economic policy. We should recall that Beveridge, while trying to cope with the circumstances of war, attempted to ease social inequality through social security and other government subsidies. Moreover, the Keynesian theory proposed to mitigate the effects of economic depression by acting on demand through the State. The implementation and further development of both conceptualizations gave rise to what we know as the Welfare State. Both right and moderate left wing political parties carried out this policy, with its most ardent defenders being the social democratic governments.

In addition, the Welfare System encouraged market and production, promoted peace, social stability and social consensus. The Welfare State has not only improved the distribution of income and affected the accumulation of capital, but has also induced changes in labour productivity, and the values and rights that were gained during an individual's lifetime. Although what we define today as a Welfare State stems from different conceptions, both philosophical and moral in their social historical genesis, the role and position of the State has been unquestioned in the epicentre of the social, economic and political process [19, 20].

Policy and legislation changes are the outcome of a negotiation process where forces and interests of the actors are confronted [21]. The process of articulation, adaptation, re-articulation, and resistance for health reforms can only be understood as valid in an economic and political context. It is particularly interesting to note that although the organized civil society and political parties usually promote changes, the State can also be involved in the negotiating process to articulate and frame changes.

Chilean Health Reforms
and Negotiation Through History

The Development
of the Welfare State

The Chilean State's efforts in the health field
began in 1890 with the creation of an agency in
charge of public hygiene and sanitation, but the
modernization of public institutions begun in
the late second and third decade of the twentieth
Century, with President Arturo Alessandri Palma.
During his first and second mandate Chile pro-
mulgated a new constitution, a new Labor Code,
Tax Law, Sanitary Law and Social Security Law,
all in anticipation of several aspects to global
trends having its origins in the treaty of Versailles
and the International Labor Organization. The
government, in pursuit of the Bismarkain example, provided health services to workers and
their families, [22, pp. 156–157] and the State
assumed an active role with universal health care
and the consolidation of State responsibility in
public health. Social security was extended for a
program that favored the employees of Railways
and the mid-20s witnessed the creation of organizations like the National Public Employees
(CANAEMPU) and the Fund for Private
Employees (EMPART).

The year 1924 (military intervention) also
marked another stage in the history of social legislation in Chile, because it was from this date
that the first social laws began to be enacted.
They were, however, welcomed by employers, workers and doctors [23]. The health legislation and reform that followed reforms were
not intended to reduce the activities of private
assistance, but to consolidate a centralized body
for social and health policies. The creation of
the Workers' Compulsory Insurance, or Social
Security, in 1924 became the central piece in the
history of public health in Chile. These events
suddenly transformed the medical profession into
a privileged intervener in the construction of the
State and radically changed the morphology of
its labor market [23]. Finally the new constitution
(1925) reflected the global trends by increasing
individual rights and the obligation of the State

in ensuring social rights, subjecting the right of
ownership to what was considered the "rule of
social progress", protecting labor and industry
and enforcing legal protection for workers and
social welfare. It also proclaimed that Public
Health Service was a duty of the State. The most
important of these social laws was the creation of
the Workers Insurance Fund, which later became
known as Social Security Service (SSS).

Later by 1938, the Popular Front Government,
(Pedro Aguirre Cerda) favorable to democratic socialist ideas, implemented the Law of
Preventive Medicine which allowed the screening of all blue and white collars workers for
contagious and chronic diseases. In 1939, Dr.
Salvador Allende, Minister of Health (who
became President in 1970), wrote a book that fur-
thered Virchow's research as he advocated that
social rather than medical solutions were necessary in order to combat current health problems.
The Chilean Socio-Medical Reality, "conceptual-
ized illness as a disturbance of the individual fos-
tered by deprived social conditions" [24, p. 75]
and focused on specific health problems that
were generated by the poor living conditions of
the working class: maternal and infant mortality,
tuberculosis and sexually transmitted diseases.

At that time these suggestions were considered
not only innovative but also definitively revolutionary. In 1940, the Popular Front Government
presented a project in which it clearly appeared
that a more comprehensive form of coverage was
needed to reduce health care inequities and centralize the management of all hospitals under a
single government agency.

The period between 1917 and 1939, patented
the State responsibility in matters of health and
welfare. However, the multiplicity of institutions
that were created resulted in costly health care service. An integrationist and centralized movement
began to develop a new alternative reform at the
end of the 30s, which reached its peak in 1952,
as a process that was developed through negotiations between governments, unions, health workers and the medical profession, each representing
its own political, economic and corporate interests [25]. The outcome was the establishment, in
1952, of the National Health Service (Servicio

Nacional de Salud—SNS), which was the major health provider in Chile for four decades. Like in Western Europe, full employment provided the ideological cement for hegemonic order throughout social democracy. In the case of Chile, the Welfare State provided the legal framework for social and health reforms, inclusive of labor protection, social stability and a more Keynesian state involvement in economic development.

Later in the 1960's, in response to pressure from the growing middle class, the government took the initiative to develop a new program for white-collar employees (SERMENA). It permitted users to select their physicians, stimulated a semi-public insurance system and created primary and preventive care clinics and laboratories for the middle class that were no longer fully covered by the public system. In this case the social sphere represented the "harmony ideology", preaching the discourse of "public interest" in order to maximize social welfare. Reforms were the culmination of an incremental process, rather than a rupture with the past, where the government was the dominant group and able to dictate reform policy over the objections of opposing interest groups in civil society [22, pp. 156–157].

As analyzed by Fleury, *"the social; policies that have developed in most Latin American countries are rooted in a similar development model. They are responsible for some of the most significant features of the relationship between the State and society, as well for the incorporation of a particular power structure into an institutionalized system"* [16, p. 1]. This pattern of structured social interactions express several characteristics, such as stratification and or exclusion of certain population groups, fragmentation of institutions, a narrow and fragile financial basis and strong actors with vested interests represented in the political arena [16, p. 1]. Health reforms were clearly "process-oriented", including the organizational structure in order to reorganize relations between public and private sectors, managers, policymakers, providers and consumers [26, p. 1].

Between 1970 and 1973, the Unidad Popular (Popular United) government introduced reforms to democratize and centralize the organizational structure of the National Health Service (SNS) [17, 27]. The government also implemented reforms to increase public involvement in health care, to control the pharmaceutical industry, to encourage citizen participation in health care management, and to achieve health care equity by creating a Unified National Health Care Service.

Hoping to resolve gaps in health benefits, the government of the *Unidad Popular* aimed to restructure health services, streamline medical care, increase access, and coordinate activities; and in turn, frame them within a dynamic and effective national plan. This task was entrusted to a Single Health Service *(Servicio Unico de Salud)*. The new organizational structure was called to incorporate public institutions and to also absorb health institutions responsible for providing health care services to the different segments of the middle class. These institutions, however, under the umbrella of the medical system for employees (SERMENA), created during the Christian Democracy government (1964–1970), alienated an important sector of the population.

This applies to the understanding that the victory of the *Unidad Popular* in Chile in 1970 cannot be considered a historical accident, but rather, the result of a crisis in the historic bloc along with the strengthening of organized popular movement. This major policy change resulted in a radicalization of the social figure of health and materialized with the completion of several transformations in this sector: a more visible presence of State control of the national pharmaceutical industry, foreign participation in the field of management and the democratization of access to services, which would lead to a unified national service. It was implemented through a health policy that ensured decisive participation of the population and the transformation of the organizational structure of the National Health Service, through centralization in decision-making and decentralization of implementation.

Although the revolutionary rhetoric was firm in place, in practical terms, these reforms did not represent a paradigm shift or a model change. They were more a change in the management of services and in the consolidation of the public sector as the spinal column and nervous center of the Chilean

Health System. It was the ultimate expression and willingness to continue with a more popular and democratic management of health services. The sum of social transformations, especially the economic transformation undertaken by the government of the *Unidad Popular* proved however to be a significant menace for large domestic and foreign economic interests.

The hegemonic shifts within the actors themselves and the role played by the State, was modifying the correlation of forces in the historical hegemonic bloc (see [28]). If the rule of law is seen as an ideology that legitimizes and conceals power relations [29, pp. 5–14], it is interesting to see how in the case of Chile, the rule of law was also instrumental for changing power relations. Thus it became clear that the other forms of power relations, like force, had to take place to reestablish bloc hegemony.

It is at this point that the breakdown of democracy appeared as a precondition for the restoration of the factors that would allow the reinstatement of the liberal economic model, earlier threatened by economic changes undertaken during the government of the *Unidad Popular*. In the field of health, the change was drastic. It altered one of the keys to Chilean social history, as the process of building the road to institutional reform in Chile (which began in the 1920s) was characterized by the legal incorporation of the working classes into the State.

The military Coup of 1973 and the restructuring of the State, which passed to play a subsidiary role, ensured the free exercise of market activities and a health market model characteristic of neo-liberal models. Incremental health reforms were disrupted by the military regime, where the implementation of a new health model, altering the previous reforms and plans, challenged the Welfare State and opened the way for a neo-liberal market model [30, 31].

The End of the Welfare State and a New Market Model

The military dictatorship (1973–1989) replaced the public-oriented system with a market-oriented approach, transferring important responsibilities to the private sector, curtailing benefits and reducing State involvement in funding of public policies and their administration [32, p. 37]. The new approaches adapted the liberal theses of economists like Rostow, Misses and Hayek and modify them to suit the final decades of the twentieth century. In Chile, this materialized in the decisive influence of the "Chicago boys" based in the University of Chicago, and particularly that of Milton Friedman and Harold Harberger. However, the state overstepped its original legal frameworks, as it intervened arbitrarily in the economy, breaking the rules of economic freedom, as it was privately criticized on several occasions by the same Milton Friedman.

The neoliberal Chicago School was opposed to governmental economic intervention, rejecting market regulations and Keynesianism and adopting monetarism, except for interventions to save the market and the banks (like in the Chilean financial crisis in the 1980s,[1] which put the new economic model in peril). The influence of this neoliberal school within the Chilean government and the particular role played by the "Chicago boys", as well as the policies of the International Monetary Fund and the World Bank, were decisive in bringing about this shift in the economic model. The new model imposed a new logic, and social consciousness around health issues became neutralized, making health concerns an individual problem and stimulating the atomization of society and the promotion of health care as business.

As already discussed, until 1973, Chile was a pioneer in Latin America in terms of social policy, developing one of the most universalistic systems on the continent. The new health model was altered in three significant areas: first, in terms of the social spending program that affected out-of-pocket spending by patient; second, by the enrollment of the middle and upper-middle class in

---

[1]The crisis in Chile that began in 1981 and lasted until 1986 saw inflation rise to almost 30% and caused a currency devaluation of 40%, which created a serious debt problem, exacerbated by a significant drop in the price of copper, the principal source of foreign exchange.

private pre-paid health institutions (ISAPRES)[2] and third, through the transfer of public health clinics to county (municipalities) management, to reduce State bureaucracy and State-financed care [33, p. 68]. These changes minimized the State's responsibilities and stimulated the development of private health care, health insurance and the growth of the pharmaceutical industry. This in turn, was a logical step for incorporating health into a liberal economic framework [34–42].

Four basic aspects of the public health care system—policy, service provision, financial management and primary care—were reorganized. Decree-Law 2763[3] (August 1979) re-organized the Ministry of Health and created the National Health Service System,[4] the National Health Fund,[5] the Public Health Institute of Chile[6] and the Central Supply Centre of the National Health

Service.[7] According to Decree-Law 2763, health service agencies were functionally de-centralized, with independent legal capacities and their own resources for fulfilling their duties. They were charged with the implementation of integrated development, protection and restoration of health and the rehabilitation of sick people. Policy-making power was transferred from the SNS back to the Ministry of Health, and the executive power to implement curative and preventive services was decentralized in the new National Health Services System.

Thirteen regions and twenty-seven semi-autonomous local health systems were created across the country, which finally became the legal successors of the National Health Service and the National Health Service for Employees (SERMENA). The health service agencies, the National Health Fund, the National Council for Food and Nutrition, the Public Health Institute of Chile, the Central Supply and the National Health Service were also brought under the ambit of the Ministry of Health[8]. The partial withdrawal of the state from curative services and the limitations suffered by the public sector in general constituted a loss of decades of progress and experience.

Social policy was guided by market-oriented principles, including the reduction of state intervention, the strengthening of the private sector, the adoption of free-market and stabilization pol icies and the privatization of public corporations

[2]Institutos de Salud Previsional, ISAPRES, created by Law 18,933 (1990) which also derogated DFL no 3 (1981).

[3]Decree Law 2763 (1979). Regulations for the Ministry of Health, National Health Service System, National Health Fund, Public Health Institute of Chile and Central Supply Centre of the National Health Service. In addition, it established the foundations for a de-regionalized National Health Care System. It established a Ministerial Health Secretariat for each of the country's regions and created Health Services authorized to delegate tasks to the universities, unions, employers' associations and other bodies with technical capacities for the activities assigned to the Health Services. The funding would come from the National Health Fund, which was the legal successor to SERMENA and the SNS.

[4]Each Service was under the charge of a director, responsible for the supervision, coordination, and control of the facilities and services of the system.

[5]The National Health Fund was a functionally de-centralized public service, with a legal capacity and financial resources of its own. Legally, it was a continuation of the National Health Service for Employees and the National Health Service, for the purpose of carrying out administrative and financial actions.

[6]The Public Health Institute of Chile was created as a functionally de-centralized public service, also with a legal capacity and financial resources of its own. It contributed to the national laboratory, and was a referential source for s the fields of Microbiology, Immunology, Pharmacology, Clinical Laboratory, Environmental Pollution and Occupational Health. It was the legal continuation of the National Health Service with respect to its relation with the Bacteriological Institute of Chile and the National Institute of Occupational Health.

[7]The Supply Center of the National Health Service came into being as a functionally de-centralized public service, again, with a legal capacity and financial resources of its own. It provided the medicines, instruments and other supplies that may be required by the agencies, organizations, institutions and persons affiliated to the Health System, for the implementation of incentive measures, protection or restoration of health, and the rehabilitation of sick people. The Supply Central was the legal successor of the National Health Service.

[8]The Ministry of Health was responsible for formulating and implementing the health policies. It had to perform the following functions: direct and guide all government activities relating to the health system; lay out the internal technical, administrative and financial regulations to be followed by the agencies, and institutions of the health system; and supervise, monitor and evaluate the implementation of policies and health plans.

and state companies and industries. Social policy had to be consistent with economic rationality [32, p. 55]. Promoting private medicine and making it profitable necessarily implied extending its market potential by increasing the consumption of private medical services. The disbursement of financial resources in the public health system was redirected from subsidizing the supply of health care services to subsidizing the demand for such services. The previous system of direct budget allocations distributed by the SNS was swapped with production criteria [43, p. 384]. Thus, the direct allocation of public funds to health care institutions via an annual budget was reduced in order to increase the allocation of funds as reimbursement for actual services rendered, creating competition between institutions. Until the sanction of Decree-Law 2575 in 1979, only 16% of the budget was allocated according to production criteria and 63.7% by direct budget allocation, with another 20% coming from direct income and donations [44]. Decree-Law 2575[9] (1979) extended the benefits of Law 16,781 to the beneficiaries of the National Health Service.

This policy of subsidizing demand even further weakened the capacity and the image of the entire public sector and stimulated the growth and legitimization of the private sector. Need-based access to services was replaced with access based on an individual's capacity to pay prices that depended on real demand as determined in a market economy, [45, p. 394] in which health care was just another commodity. The "demand" for health care was not actually the result of an individual's decision to use medical services based on his or her medical needs; rather, it was the result of several other factors, such as

the capacity to pay and the accessibility of services [46, pp. 31–32]. Additional factors taken into consideration by patients included the subsequent cost of follow-up treatments and drugs[10] as well as the loss of income during recovery. Given these constraints, which were not insignificant, increasing the capacity of patients and users to pay became one of the financial challenges of the new liberal health care model. This situation was further exacerbated when the principles of cooperation and coordination between different services and institutions were replaced with inter-institutional competition. There was also a tendency to reorganize the availability of services to target the most profitable types of medical specializations.

The goal was to facilitate the transfer of savings to private insurance institutions, thus increasing the users' capacity to choose services and simultaneously stimulating the private practice of medicine and the development of private clinics and, eventually, hospitals. The new market approach was clearly reflected in the type and variety of services offered, which now had to incorporate time as a variable to maximize profit. Furthermore, artificial demand was created with the introduction of more screening appointments, excess consumption of non-essential medical services and the promotion of greater drug use, all

---

[9]Decree-Law 2575 extended the medical and dental benefits of Law 16,781 (1968) to the beneficiaries of the National Health Service. The legal beneficiaries of the National Health Service were eligible for the health care system under Law 16,781, without prejudice to the care that they were entitled to of that service in accordance with Law 10,383 and its amendments. The National Health Service had to pay the amount equal to the percentage paid by the Medical Assistance Fund, as established by Law 16,781. Any difference between the amount funded by the National Health Service and the total value of the benefit was charged to the beneficiary.

---

[10]In developed countries, drug expenses represented between 9% and 10% of the budget destined for health services. These figures more than doubled in underdeveloped countries. These numbers were even more eloquent in Chile, as it was reported that pharmaceutical expenses comprised of almost a third of all expenses recorded in the health sector. Ernesto Medina & Ana María, Kaempfer, "Análisis crítico de la metodología de planificación de salud", (1968) *Revista Médica de Chile 455*. The concentration of the pharmaceutical industry in Chile demonstrated that in 1977, out of 57 active companies, 24 were foreign and the 5 largest of these already controlled 32% of the market. The leading 25 companies controlled 80.5% of the total market and 18 were foreign multinationals. Also, since foreign pharmaceutical companies hold patents rights the possibility of transfer of technologies was very limited. At the same time, this allowed artificially high pricing, sales linked to the purchase of other products and finally restrictions in domestic exportation. See Constantine Vaitsos in Meredeth Turshen, "An analysis of the medical supply industries", (1976) *6 International Journal of Health Services* at 275.

part of, as described by the regime, a sophisticated approach to medical care.

The privatization process was based on a very clear economic rationale of stating why and how to impose and implement the new liberal market model in the health sector, which, as indicated above, included an articulated process to reduce the public sector, stimulate the growth of the private sector and lastly, expand the market for the private sector. This was precisely in line with neoliberal political and economic principles, according to which private sector interests and market laws become the impulse for development. In summary, these political-economic policies in the health field were no guarantee of better health care; rather, they were tools to increase the profitability of the "business" of medicine and the medical-industrial complex.

These clearly neo-liberal reforms changed the relationship between State and society, either by replacing political logic with market principles or by creating new forms of control and participation [47, pp. 27–28]. International financial institutions have played, and continue to play a significant role in the formation of social policy, particularly in areas of health and pension programs. Social security reforms have been promoted by the World Bank loans under a neo-liberal framework, in which the market becomes responsible for providing health and pensions. The neo-liberal reforms were able to start the dismantling of the Welfare State, where the State became only responsible for the poor. However with limited financial resources this can only mean limited access and care [48].

Although these reforms were presented as an appropriate strategy for the rationalization and modernization of the health care system (as it was believed to improve efficiency and effectiveness, while reducing cost and bureaucracy), they were criticized for both their inequities and their prioritization of market expansion [31, 42, 49, 50].

We must look to the history of Chilean society and its profound inequalities to understand why the majority of the population was unable to exercise this "freedom option". The government initially believed that the real freedom of individuals would be guaranteed by the subsidiary role of the state, as individual and personal relations with curative services would be strengthened. To privatize social security and to alter the responsibility of the state in the services sector meant to transform "social concern" into an "individual concern". This change was also politically interesting given the traditional strength of the health sector as a force of organization and popular cohesion.

It is, in effect, with respect to health issues that people may develop a "social consciousness" about the problems that afflict individuals. This consciousness allows them to share similar claims and channel forms of social struggle. Castells and Clarke [51, 52, p. 102] defines these processes of politicization as a "socialization of claims" where collective consciousness focuses on collective action. In contrast, the neutralization of claims and the atomization of society stem precisely from the individualization of interests, when health issues become individual problems and not social concerns. This particular scenario also echoed the global health care crisis, characterized by fiscal limitations for the expansion of socialized medicine in increasingly expensive health care scenarios. In the face of the increasing cost of care and the significant financial impacts of chronic diseases that accompany an aging population, the high demand for pharmaceuticals and more demanding specialized technology, reforms and potential solutions focused mainly on organizational and financial measures to contain costs, improve efficiency and transfer the responsibility to patients. The crisis of modern, specialized medicine, accelerated by demographic and epidemiological transitions, was also revealing how the patient was becoming the target to blame in the health-illness process [53, p. 663] and the source of revenue in the health care business.

As discussed the military regime established a new legal framework that redefined the public system, creating open competition between medical establishments. According to promoters of the model, this new "healthy and effective competition in health care services" was a correction to the state's ineffectiveness as a provider of medical services and a solution for the "financial anarchy" of distributing resources and establishing costs [54]. They reiterated that the reform process not only imposed regulations on the public sector to improve its effectiveness, but also brought renewed economic dynamism to the management of curative services, which would result in "increased income for health professionals", "more new sources of employment", "a new incentive to the investment-deprived sector" and "reduced health costs" [55].

However, despite the government's principles and objectives, transformations in the health sector were not easy to implement and did not take place as quickly as expected. Although supporters of the model continued to try to implement a broad, market-driven approach, others within the same military regime were more cautious and preferred to keep the state as the principal actor responsible for the health sector. The internal dissent and conflicts between health professionals slowed down the Ministry's action plans and brought modifications to the proposed health model. The public sector had historically been considered to play a fundamental role in health care, with a role too critically important to be suddenly modified. Thus, the government was forced to continuously defend itself from its critics, indicating that it did not want to implement "either a cold market model or a state model". Its polemical pragmatic discourse favoured a combination of market policies and policies based on the responsibility of the state. The regime labelled it a "social market economy", probably following the liberal German model. The idea was that the private sector and the market would invigorate social development, while the subsidiary role of the state would protect fundamental social interests.

After the years of dictatorship and when the Pinochet regime was later replaced by the democratic Aylwin government in 1989, the country saw an establishment of new changes and reforms; particularly a renewal of State intervention and implication in the Health field. Rather than a complete withdrawal from previous reforms, this however was accomplished progressively [22, p. 165; 12, p. 372], since the hegemonic bloc that had its roots in the authoritarian period was still politically influential within a framework of electoral democracy [12, p. 372].

One of the major consequences of the changing role of the State in health policy has been the blurring of the respective roles, responsibilities and jurisdictions of the public and private spheres [56]. Today, in Chile, the health services system can be labeled as a "mixed system", through its combinational financing and service provision. In the current context of liberalization of a globalized economy and of fiscal inability to assume all costs of benefits, it is virtually impossible to imagine a return to the Welfare State, or to dramatically reverse the privatization processes. Also, it shall be recognized that the growing, so called, middle class, often caught between a public sector with enormous difficulties to satisfy their health care needs along with their own economic capacity to resort to private medicine, have benefited from the extending private health insurances. Consecutive Chilean governments under the administration of the center-left political coalitions (first the *Concertación por la Democracia and later the Nueva Mayoría*), elected and reelected in five elections, following the end of the dictatorship, have made progressive but not radical changes in health policies. These governments maintained the foundations of the model, but progressively implemented reforms to expand coverage, improve the public system, and allow for major investments in health infrastructure, which illustrates that health policies and reforms are not only the outcome of economic and political change, but also the result of negotiations between different players.

Conclusion

The State apparatus has always had enormous importance in the structure and administration of Chilean society and has even assumed a leading role since the second half of the twentieth century. The State has penetrated corners of public and private social life, becoming the most important agent of production and reproduction of society.

An adequate study of the whole cannot be developed from the separate study of individual parts. Legislation and legal institutions have a dialectic and constitutive relationship to the socio-economic political structure. Therefore, healthcare reforms should be situated within a larger context to enable the examination of the relationship between social reforms, economic structure, and political variables in a given historical context.

Health reforms and changes to a particular historical context are the result of a negotiation and articulation of different interests in a dynamic hegemony. In this process a number of interrelated factors and variables come into play, power is exercised and hegemonies are established. The negotiation process for health legislation and health changes, historically implemented in Chile were the result of political and economic choices, motivated by various ideologies, and mediated by a diversity of actors (e.g. professionals, health workers, the general public and private interests).

Changes in health have been spiraling where and when political parties, federations of trade unions and the organized civil society have prompted transformations and applied strength and pressure to legislate in the area of health. The formulation of public policy on health does not result in the imposition of one group over the rest, but rather in the articulation of interests and ideologies of one class in relation to the rest of society. In essence, this scenario allows for an understanding of the by-play interests which lead to major changes in health reforms as well as an understanding of the negotiation process between a web of economic, political and social forces.

References

1. Murdock CJ. Physicians, the state and public health in Chile, 1881-1891. J Lat Am Stud. 1995;27(3):551–67.
2. Trumper R, Phillips L. Give me discipline and give me death: neoliberalism and health in Chile. Race and Class. 1996;37(Jan/Mar):19–34.
3. Frenk J. Dimensions of health system reform. Health Policy. 1994;27:19–34.
4. Fitzpatrick T. In search of a welfare democracy. Soc Policy Soc. 2002;1(1):11–20.
5. Poulantzas N. Political power and social class. London: New Left Books; 1973; Joseph J. A realist theory of hegemony. J Theory Soc Behav. 2000; 30(2):188. (Blackwell Publishers, Oxford).
6. Althusser L, Balibar E. Reading capital (trans: Brewster, B.). New Left Books. 1965.
7. Gramsci A. Selection of the Prison Notebooks. London: Lawrence and Wisharts; 1971; Joseph J. A realist theory of hegemony. J Theory Soc Behav. 2000; 30(2): 181. (Blackwell Publishers, Oxford).
8. Gill S. Epistemology, ontology and the 'Italian School. In: Gill S, editor. Gramsci, historical materialism and international relations. Cambridge Univ. Press; 1993; Barrios P. Liberal environmentalism and the international law of hazardous chemicals. Ph.D. Dissertation, University of British Columbia. 2007. p. 21.
9. Rupert M. Alienation, capitalism and the inter-state system: towards a Marxian/Gramscian critique. In: Gill S, editor. Gramsci, historical materialism and international relations. Cambridge Univ. Press; 1993; Barrios P. Liberal environmentalism and the international law of hazardous chemicals. Ph.D. Dissertation, University of British Columbia; 2007. p. 21.
10. Augelli E, Murphy C. America's quests for supremacy and the third world: a Gramscian analysis. London: Pinter in Rupert Mark; 1993.
11. Joseph J. A realist theory of hegemony. J Theory Soc Behav. 2000;30(2):179–202. (Blackwell Publishers, Oxford, UK)
12. Barton J. State Continuismo and Pinochetismo: The Keys to Chilean transition. Bull Lat Am Res. 2002;21(3):358–74.
13. Eldabi T, Irani Z, Paul RJ. A proposed approach for modeling health care systems for understanding. J Manag Med. 2002; 16(2/3): 170–187; Gómez CA. Influencia de los grupos de interés. Revista Gerencia y Políticas de Salud. No 9, December 2005.
14. CIESS, Conferencia Interamericana de Seguridad Social. Informe anual sobre la seguridad social en las Américas 2005. Fragmentación y alternativas para aumentar la cobertura del seguro en dalud, Mexico, DF. 2004; Gómez CA. Influencia de los grupos de interés. Revista Gerencia y Políticas de Salud. 2005; No 9, December, 2005.
15. Heidenheimer A, et al. Comparative public policy. New York: St.Martin's Press; 1990.
16. Fleury S. Reforming health care in Latin America: challenges and options. In: Fleury S, Belmartino S, Baris E, editors. Reshaping health care in Latin America, Chap. 1. Ottawa: IDRC; 2000.
17. Tedeschi SK, Brown TM, et al. Salvador Allende: physician, socialist, populist, and president. J Public Health. 2003;93(12):2014–5.
18. Gómez CA. Influencia de los grupos de interés y asociación en las reformas y los sistemas de salud. Gerencia y Políticas de Salud. 2005;9:62–80.

19. Picó, J. Modelos sobre el Estado de Bienestar. De la ideología a la práctica. In: Casilda R, Tortosa, J. editors. Pros y contras del Bienestar, Madrid: Tecnos; 1966; Parada M. Ph.D. Dissertation, Universidad Autónoma de Madrid, Spain, 2004.

20. Picó J. Teorías sobre el Estado del Bienestar. Madrid: Siglo Veintiuno de España Editores; 1999; Parada M. Ph.D. Dissertation, Universidad Autónoma de Madrid, Spain, 2004.

21. Ratliff W. Development and civil society in Latin America and Asia. Ann Am Acad Political Soc Sci. 1999;565(1):91–112.

22. de la Jiménez Jara J, Bossert T. Chile's health sector reform: lessons from four reform periods. Health Policy. 1995;32:155–66.

23. Parada M. Ph.D. Dissertation, Universidad Autónoma de Madrid, Spain, 2004.

24. Waitzkin H, Iriart C, Estrada A, Lamadrid S. Social medicine then and now: lessons from Latin America. Am J Public Health. 2001;91:1592–601.

25. Belmar R, et al. Teaching of public health and social medicine. Rev Méd Chil. 1971;99(7):529–35.

26. Horev T, Babad Y. Healthcare reform implementation: stakeholders and their roles – the Israeli experience. Health Policy. 2005;71:1–21.

27. de la Jiménez Jara J, editor. Medicina Social en Chile. Santiago: Ediciones Aconcagua; 1977.

28. Barrios P. Liberal environmentalism and the international law of hazardous chemicals. Ph.D Dissertation, University of British Columbia; 2007.

29. Unger RM. The critical legal studies movement. Cambridge: Harvard University Press; 1993.

30. Chossudovsky M. Human rights, health and capital accumulation en the third world. Int J Health Serv. 1979;9(1):61–75.

31. Taylor M. The Reformulation of Social Policy in Chile, 1973-2001. Questioning a Neoliberal Model. Glob Soc Policy. 2003;3(1):21–44.

32. Castiglioni R. The politics of retrenchment: the quandaries of social protection under military rule in Chile, 1973-1990. Lat Am Politics Soc. 2001;43(4):37–66.

33. Scarpaci JL, Bradham DD. A three-tiered health system and its inherent cost inflation: the case of medical care inflation in Chile 1979-1983. Health Policy. 1988;10:65–76.

34. Bravo A. Sistemas y modelos de Organización de Salud. In: Lavados H, editor. Desarrollo Social y Salud en Chile, (first part). Santiago: Corporación de Promoción Universitaria; 1980.

35. Bruce N. The chilean health care reforms: model or myth? J Publ Int Aff. 2000;11:69–86.

36. Ehrenreich B, Ehrenreich J. The American health empire: power, profits, and politics. New York: Random House; 1970.

37. Flaño N. Planificación o mercado en el sector salud enfoque teórico con aplicación al caso de Chile, Apuntes CIEPLAN, No 19, October, 1979.

38. Livingstone M. In: Raczinsky D, editor. Salud Pública y Bienestar Social. Santiago: CIEPLAN; 1976.

39. Ministerio de Salud. Política Económica y financiamiento de la salud. October, 1979.

40. Nocvak V. The other drug lords. Int J Health Serv. 1993;23(2):263–73.

41. Ruderman P. Economic adjustment and the future of health services in the Third World. J Public Health Policy. 1990;11(4):481–90.

42. Sapelli C. Risk segmentation and equity in the Chilean mandatory health insurance system. Soc Sci Med. 2004;58(2):259–65.

43. Viveros-Long AM. Changes in the health financing: the Chilean experience. Soc Sci Med. 1986;22:384.

44. Bize R. Asignación de Recursos Financieros a las regiones de Salud y Sistema de Costos Hospitalarios in Lavados, Desarrollo Social y Salud en Chile. In: Montes L, editor. Desarrollo Social y Salud en Chile. Santiago: Corporación de Promoción Universitaria; 1981. p. 382; Viveros-Long A. Changes in the health financing: the Chilean experience. Soc Sci Med. 1986; 22: 394.

45. Bravo AB. Principios básicos para la organización de un sistema de servicios de salud: el caso chileno. In: Lavados Desarrollo Social y Salud en Chile. Ibid; 1980. p. 394.

46. De Kadt E. Las desigualdades en el campo de la salud. In: Livingstone, Raczynski, editors. Salud Pública y Bienestar Social. Santiago: CIEPLAN; 1976. p. 31–2.

47. Fleury S. Reshaping health care in Latin America: toward fairness? In: Fleury S, Belmartino S, Baris E, editors. Reshaping Health Care in Latin America, Chap. 9. Ottawa: IDRC; 2000.

48. Berlinguer G. Globalization and global health. Int J Health Serv. 1999;29(3):579–95.

49. Isaacs S, Solimano G. Health reform and civil society in Latin America. Development. 1999;42(4):70–2.

50. Kay SJ. The perils of private pensions. Foreign Policy. 2000;118:21.

51. Castells M. Análisis marxista de la crisis del capitalismo. In: Mercer H, Escudero JC, editors. Políticas de Salud en los Estados capitalistas de excepción: Argentina, Chile y Uruguay. México: UAM-Xochimilco, Editorial Mimeo; 1979.

52. Clarke DB. Consumer society and the post-modern city. New York: Routledge; 2003.

53. Crawford R. You are dangerous to your health: the ideology and politics of victim blaming. Int J Health Serv. 1977;7:663.

54. El Mercurio. Editorials 2, 6, 10 & 22 May, 1981.

55. El Mercurio. Editorials 8 & 29 May, 1981.

56. Cutler, et al. In: Buse K, Dagerk N, Fustukian S, Lee K, editors. Globalisation and health policy trends and opportunities; Lee K, et al. editors. Health politics in a globalasing world, Cambridge University Press; 2001. p. 253. 1999.

Prasad Godbole and Derek Burke

Introduction

Who Are Medical Leaders?

Historically non-clinical managers managed hospitals with clinicians providing front line services [1]. Over the decades, more and more clinicians have taken on managerial responsibility and in many instances giving up their clinical duties to take on full time management roles. In the US a recent survey has shown that up to 51% of managers in hospitals are doctors [2].

In countries such as India, hospitals may be as small as 5–10 beds and owned and managed by doctors in their entirety. Larger corporate hospitals with up to 2000 beds are managed jointly by doctors and non-clinical managers. A systematic review has shown some evidence to suggest that where doctors work in a hybrid role as clinicians and managers, the performance of the hospital is better than for hospitals having only non-clinical managers [3]. Such findings often give rise to heated debate and can lead to polarised views. Many people argue that doctors in managerial roles may not have the necessary expertise or experience in management to run highly complex organisations and could be biased by their clinical views in terms of hospital innovation and transformation. Others argue that doctors prefer to be led by doctors and the role of the medical manager acts as a conduit between the hospital board and the shop floor. A third view suggests that where medical managers continue to provide direct clinical care to patients, they will tend to prioritise their clinical responsibilities rather than their managerial responsibilities thereby putting undue additional pressure on their management colleagues, often at critical times such as the winter period.

Whatever the arguments for and against medical managers, it is clear that greater numbers of doctors are venturing into management roles but at the same time retaining at least some of their clinical responsibilities. Increasingly doctors are gaining qualifications in medical leadership and healthcare management thereby increasing their understanding of the management process. The gaining of such qualifications addresses some of the perceived experiential gap between professional non-clinical managers and emerging clinician managers.

Wider Context

For any hospital to succeed, the hospital as a whole must have a vision that the entire organisational staff signs up to. To achieve this corporate

P. Godbole (✉)
Department of Paediatric Surgery, Sheffield
Children's NHS Foundation Trust, Sheffield, UK
e-mail: Prasad.Godbole@sch.nhs.uk

D. Burke
Department of Emergency Medicine, Sheffield
Children's NHS Foundation Trust, Sheffield, UK
e-mail: Derek.Burke@sch.nhs.uk

© Springer Nature Switzerland AG 2019

D. Burke et al. (eds.), *Hospital Transformation*, https://doi.org/10.1007/978-3-030-15448-6_9

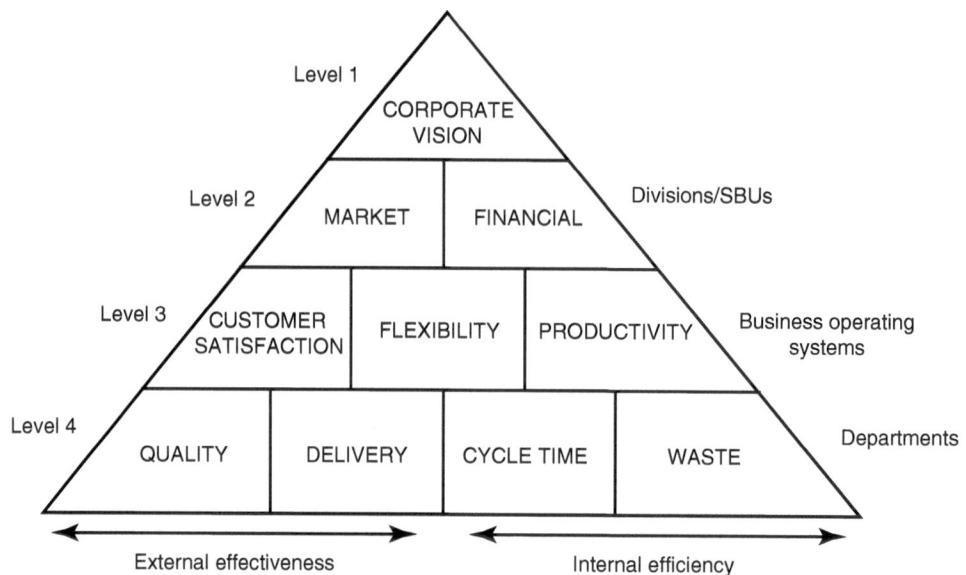

Fig. 9.1 Project management triangle. Source Lynch and Cross 1989 (http://erepository.uonbi.ac.ke/bitstream/handle/11295/100103/Kamau_Performance%20 Measurement%20Practices%20and%20Operational%20 Performance%20of%20Manufacturing%20Firms%20 in%20Kenya.pdf?sequence=1&isAllowed=y)

vision, the management team must understand the cost of providing the services and how the vision can be delivered within the organisational cost ceiling. Customer (patient) satisfaction must be monitored and minimum productivity standards agreed with the flexibility to increase productivity as necessary. Finally with productivity comes the quality of service delivery and outcomes and the minimising of waste. The above project management triangle (Fig. 9.1) can be simplified for healthcare organisations as shown below:

For any hospital to function requires a specified operating budget for the day to day operations of the hospital including staff salaries, equipment, procurement, maintenance etc. The performance of the hospital is the activities the hospital undertakes to generate income. This productivity in turn has to be balanced by the quality of outcomes, patient experience and patient safety. With increasing constraints on healthcare resource allocation may it be in insured/private markets or those free at the point of delivery, management teams must maintain the delicate balance between the three factors. Where performance and productivity reduces, this generates

less revenue with less money to be spent on cleanliness of the hospital or quality improvement programs. In the US, this has led to some hospitals having their Joint Committee Accreditation revoked or Medicaid/Medisure contracts terminated. In the U.K. the National Health Service Hospitals are monitored across a number of patient focused domains for the quality of care (Care Quality Commission)[1] and financial viability also scrutinised by MONITOR[2]—a governmental regulatory body.

How Can Medical Leaders Assist in the Turnaround Process?

As already discussed previously, more and more doctors are leaning towards management roles in an executive capacity. In the U.K. there is a hierarchical organisational management structure with medical representation at executive board level. A generic outline of the management

---

[1] www.cqc.org.uk.

[2] https://improvement.nhs.uk/resources/?publishingbody= monitor.

Fig. 9.2 The inverted pyramid

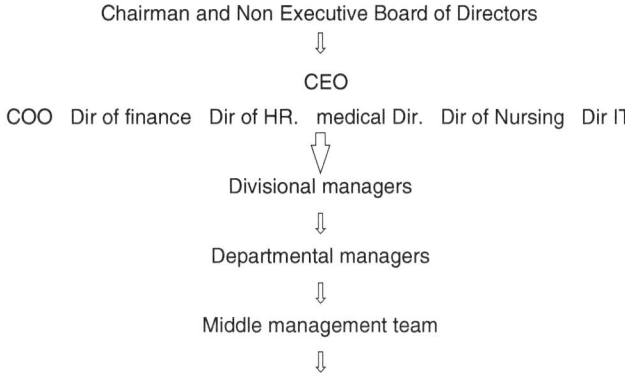

Chairman and Non Executive Board of Directors
⇩
CEO

COO   Dir of finance   Dir of HR.   medical Dir.   Dir of Nursing   Dir IT
⇩
Divisional managers
⇩
Departmental managers
⇩
Middle management team
⇩
Doctors, nurses, allied healthcare workers, non clinical staff

structure is shown below As can be seen from the above, there is a tendency for a top down approach with the 'doers' at the bottom of the pyramid and the decision makers at the top- an inverted pyramid (Fig. 9.2).

Background

The medical director approaches a transformational change process in a hospital with trepidation. The hospital will be under significant scrutiny and may have external consultants directing the day to day activity and expenditure of the hospital. The medical director will be under considerable pressure to contribute to the delivery of financial savings but should be clear about their prime professional responsibility which is to ensure that patients are safe. Before describing an approach to this task we need to understand the strategic landscape in which hospitals operate and the inter-relationship between cost, quality, safety and risk.

Strategic Objectives of Hospitals

In addition to any internal strategic objectives all hospitals have three common strategic objectives:

1. Finance: staying within budget
2. Delivery: delivering a volume of activity sufficient to generate sufficient income to ensure

a balanced budget and at the same time meet targets
3. Experience: ensuring patients are receiving good quality, safe care

We use the term quality here to meet delivering to standard, e.g. if the standard is one qualified nurse to every four patients then delivering that level of cover meets the criteria for achieving the quality standard for nursing levels. Falling below this level means that the quality standard has not been met. If the standard is evidence based then failure to meet that standard is likely to increase the risk to patient safety.

Finance, Delivery and Experience are inter-related. Hospitals need to deliver sufficient activity to generate income to remain in financial balance and meet targets to avoid financial difficulties or even regulatory penalties. Hospitals require sufficient income to recruit and retain staff to deliver activity and maintain a safe, high quality service. Hospitals have to achieve all three at the same time.

Organisations run into problems when there is undue focus on one strategic objective to the detriment of the other two: commonly a disproportionate focus on financial stability at the expense of delivery and experience. Because of the inter-relationship between cost, quality and safety a failure to balance the three strategic objectives will inevitably results in compromised patient safety.

As the diagram below (Fig. 9.3) indicates it is the function of the Hospital Senior Management

Fig. 9.3 Inter-relationship between
cost, quality, safety and risk

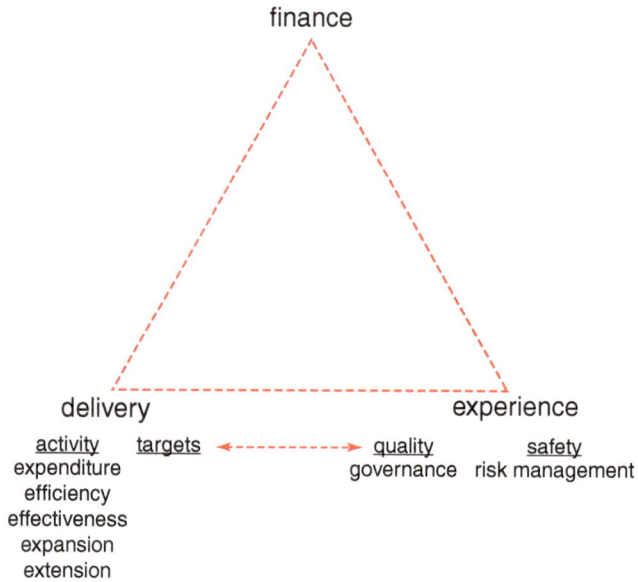

Fig. 9.4 Interrelationship between
cost, quality and safety

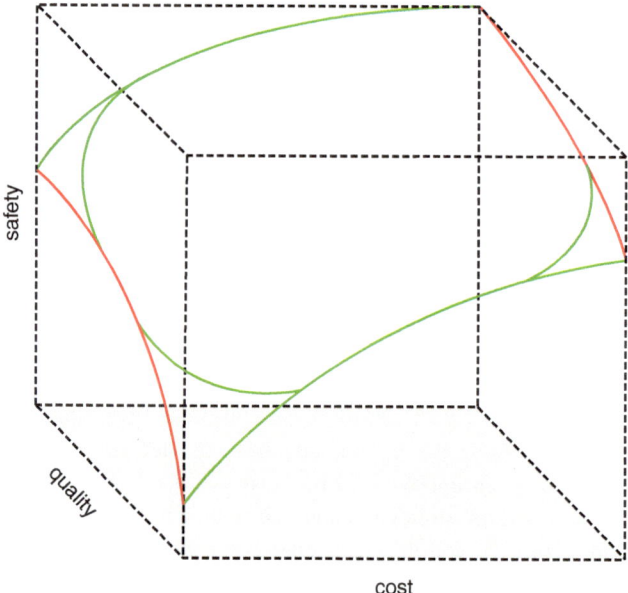

Team to ensure that the three objectives are given
equitable consideration.

Hospitals spend money in order to deliver
high quality activity safely. Ensuring there is sufficient staffing of the right level of experience and
skill mix to deliver services is the major item of
expenditure for most hospitals (~75% of the average hospital expenditure in the UK). Money
(Cost) is expended to deliver specified aspects of

care to agreed standards (Quality) to ensure that
patients are kept form harm (Safe). The following
graph (Fig. 9.4) provides a qualitative representation of the inter-relationship.

A minimum level of expenditure is required to
deliver a given level of safety. For each level of
expenditure there is a range of levels of safety
which can be realised depending on the decisions
on what money is spent on. The wrong decision

on what to spend money will realise a lower level of safety for a given expenditure than is possible.

We can describe the three dimension surface (Fig. 9.5) which the cost/quality/safety matrix maps out as the patient safety landscape. High levels of expenditure generally result in a safe environment in which the organisation is regulated but at arm's length (as long as the metrics used to assess the organisation's safety profile are maintained). A low level of expenditure is more likely to result in a less safe environment: in extreme cases the hospital may be put into spe-

cial measures or have significant restrictions by the regulators. But note that judicious decision making by an organisation with lower expenditure due to financial constraints can still be associated with a safe environment.

Note that this landscape illustrates a qualitative model for the relationship between cost/quality and safety. We can add a quantitative element by mapping out the hospital's incident risk scores onto the landscape. This is illustrated below for a hospital which is low risk (Fig. 9.6). The validity of this mapping is predicted on a good reporting culture which can be assessed by the position of

Fig. 9.5 Patient safety landscape as a three dimension surface

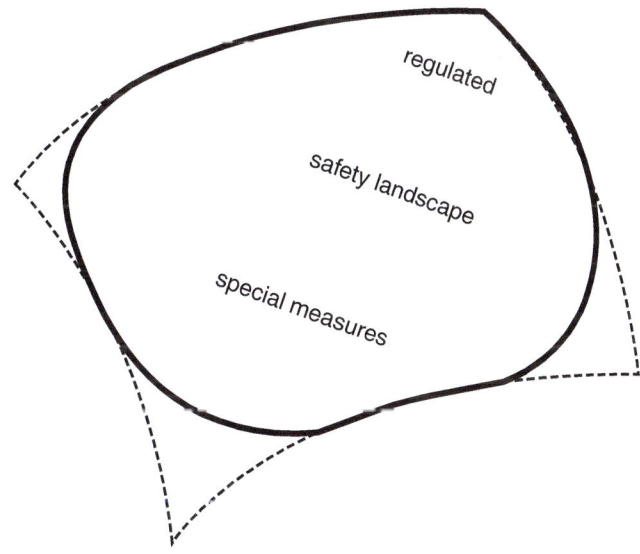

Fig. 9.6 Mapping of incident scores of a low risk hospital on patient safety landscape

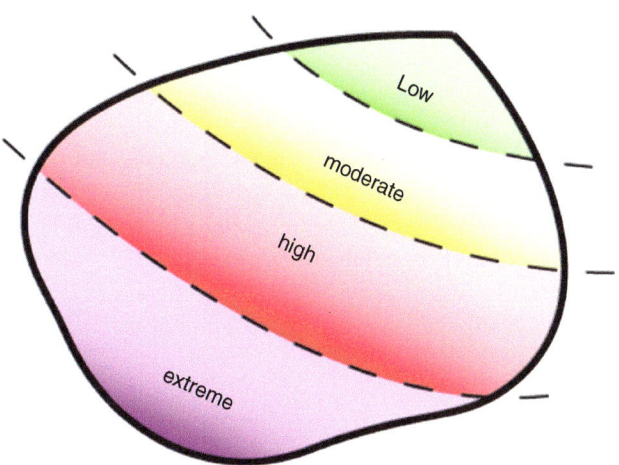

the organisation on the reporting metric chart for example on the National Reporting and Learning System site for Hospitals in England.[3]

The Medical Director in a Failing Hospital Undergoing Transformation

The medical director must be able to differentiate between the important priorities and the urgent priorities. Urgent patient safety issues will need to be addressed as they arise. The important priorities are less time dependant but there will be pressure to prioritise them as they will usually relate to primary finance issues (cutting costs) or secondary finance issues (ensuring income is secured through the maintenance of activity levels).

In addressing the important problems the medical director should allow themselves sufficient time to run a thorough diagnostic on the hospital. In the best of times this process can take upwards of 3 months (ask any medical director how long it took them to gain an understanding of the issues in their new job and they will rarely come up with a figure of less than 3 months). For a hospital in turnaround the same timescale should be adhered to. Failure to undertake an accurate diagnostic analysis will have similar consequences to arriving at the wrong diagnosis in a patient: at best time wasted pursuing solutions which will not work; at worse causing harm to patients.

The medical director will be pressurised to find solutions to the problem with the risk that they will generate solutions without clearly identifying the underlying problems: identifying the root cause of the failure is a pre-requisite to coming up with solutions. It is often the case that when the true problems have been identified the correct solutions present themselves.

Do not be rushed into arriving at pre-emptive solutions until you are sure you are aware of the underlying problems. Overall this will lead to a longer time required to bring the organisation back into a sustainable position.

When running the diagnostic three parallel tracks should be pursued:

A review of the papers of the last three Hospital board, board committees and corporate management team meetings will give an insight into the managerial function of the organisation from the management perspective.

Walking the floor to speak with the frontline staff who delivers the service is crucial. They will inform the medical director of the front line staff's perspective of the management culture and its impact on the quality and safety within the organisation. Staff will usually be aware of the key operational issues which need addressing.

The patient's perspective can be assessed by speaking with patients who are currently using the service and by reviewing complaints, Serious Incident Root Cause Analyses and patient surveys (in-patient, out-patient and the emergency department).

Needless to say the staff and patients will give the medical director the best insight into the effectiveness of the management team. Trends in the staff survey should form a key part of this review.

The review of the minutes of the committees, staff and patient perspective will usually provide sufficient information for the medical director to ascertain the core problems within the hospital and to formulate solutions.

The next stage is to develop a strategy to address the problems. The early wins will be achieved by addressing workforce health and wellbeing issues and reviewing the organisation's values set and how well they have been implemented. A rapid assessment of whether the information being acted on is based on accurate and timely data collection, submission and analysis is essential. As quantitative finance data and information is usually easy to collate there is a risk that this will be prioritised; do not underestimate the value and power of qualitative data and information. Staff and patients views,

---

[3] https://improvement.nhs.uk/resources/learning-from-patient-safety-incidents/.

properly triangulated will provide earlier warnings of patient safety going off track than the quantitative data provided in board reports.

The early diagnostic phase is likely to take up to 3 months: it can be achieved in less but time will inevitably be taken up in managing urgent operational issues which are directly threatening patient safety. This diagnostic will generally suggest the strategy to be followed, the priority to be assigned to the individual components of the strategy and a realistic timescale for the individual actions.

References

1. Spehar I, Frich JC, Kjekshus LE. Clinicians in management: a qualitative study of managers' use of influence strategies in hospitals. BMC Health Serv Res. 2014;14:251.
2. Clay-Williams R, Ludlow K, Testa L, Li Z, Braithwaite J. Medical leadership, a systematic narrative review: do hospitals and healthcare organisations perform better when led by doctors? BMJ Open. 2017;7(9):e014474.
3. Sarto F, Veronesi G. Clinical leadership and hospital performance: assessing the evidence base. BMC Health Serv Res. 2016;16(Suppl 2):169.

Erwin Loh and Katherine Lorenz

About This Chapter

This chapter sets out a proposed public health service's governance framework and describes the systems in place to ensure that the health service Board, Executive and all staff of the organisation are accountable for the clinical, corporate, financial and operational aspects of the organisation.

Good Governance Provides the Foundation for High Performance

Good governance strengthens community confidence in public entities and helps ensure their reputations are maintained and enhanced. It should enable public entities to perform efficiently and effectively and to respond strategically to changing demands.

Governance encompasses the processes by which public entities are directed, controlled and held to account. It includes the processes whereby decisions important to the future of a public entity are taken, communicated, monitored and assessed.

Governance in the public sector is built on:

- constitutional, legal and government frameworks;
- government decision making and reporting;
- authorisations and delegations in decision-making;
- accountability, transparency, integrity, stewardship, efficiency and leadership;
- values and codes of conduct;
- effective risk management;
- the integrity bodies—protecting public entities against crime and misconduct.

A board with decision-making powers is formed to govern a public entity. Governance gives practical meaning to public sector accountability obligations. For such public entities, governance defines the relationships between the board, senior management, the minister, portfolio department, stakeholders and integrity bodies.

Victorian Public Sector Commissioner[1]

E. Loh (✉) · K. Lorenz
Monash Centre for Health Research
and Implementation, Monash University,
Clayton, VIC, Australia
e-mail: erwin.loh@monash.edu; ceo@vicbar.com.au

[1] https://vpsc.vic.gov.au/governance/governance-structure-and-roles/governance-structure/.

© Springer Nature Switzerland AG 2019
D. Burke et al. (eds.), *Hospital Transformation*, https://doi.org/10.1007/978-3-030-15448-6_10

Case Study

The public health service in question is one of the largest public health services in Australia, which provided healthcare to one quarter of this state's population, across the entire life-span from newborn and children, to adults, the elderly, their families and carers. The health service has more than 17,000 staff work at over 40 care locations, including six hospital campuses, and an extensive network of rehabilitation, aged care, community health and mental health facilities.

Each year, the health service provided more than 3.6 million episodes of care to its community, with more than 260,000 people admitted to its hospitals, more than 220,000 receiving care at its emergency departments, performing more than 48,000 surgical procedures, and delivering more than 10,000 babies.

The health service for many years did not have a consolidated governance framework that was clearly articulated in a single document located centrally that was easily accessible to its staff, patients and the community. As a result, there was confusion as to the role of the health service Board, its Executive team, the senior managers and the frontline staff. This led to a confused delegation of authority leading to unclear lines of accountability, a lack of discipline around financial management, poor procurement practices, uncoordinated and unrestricted staff appointments, and disjointed reporting lines, which resulted in an adverse budget outcome due to uncontrolled costs, uncapped staff increases and lack of contract management, as well as low staff morale from reactive actions taken by middle managers to attempt to compensate for the poor governance.

A review occurred with the appointment of new executives, including a new Chief Legal Officer, which led to a systematic review and the development of a new governance framework from the ground-up, which included clear delineation of roles and responsibilities of all levels of management and staff, that are evidence-based, compliant with legislation and accessible to all employees.

The result of this is an almost immediate improvement in staff morale and culture as there were now clearly lines of accountability and reporting, with a concomitant improvement in financial outcomes, procurement practices and overall better clinical, operational and budget performance. The case study shows the importance of starting with the foundation of the principles of good, robust governance, and how that forms the basis of effective health service provision that leads to great patient care and an excellent staff and patient experience.

This chapter provides a template for other public health services who may wish to embark on a similar journey of developing their own governance framework and includes a check-list that may be helpful as part of that process.

Health Service Clinical Governance

Clinical Governance is a systematic and integrated approach to assurance and review of clinical responsibility and accountability that improves quality and safety and patient outcomes.[2] Clinical Governance is linked to corporate governance, strategic risk and service planning, informatics, performance and business management. The Health Service Clinical Governance Framework is the system by which the Board, Executive, clinicians and staff share responsibility and accountability for the safety and quality of care. Clinicians and clinical teams are responsible and accountable for the quality of care provided. The Board and Executive are responsible and accountable for ensuring the systems, structures and processes are in place to support clinicians in providing safe, high quality care and for clinician engagement in improvement and risk management activities.

Compliance of clinical governance is measured through accreditation mechanisms and through the health service Quality Committee

---

[2] https://www.safetyandquality.gov.au/wp-content/uploads/2017/11/National-Model-Clinical-Governance-Framework.pdf.

which provides leadership and advice to the Board through the continuous assessment and evaluation of the safety and quality of clinical services provided by health service.

Corporate and Financial Governance

The Board needs to meet a range of requirements under the relevant financial legislation; including keeping proper financial accounts, risk management, audit arrangements, financial reporting, annual reporting to Parliament and responding to Ministerial requests for information.

To comply with the obligations in the relevant financial legislation, the public health service must ensure that, inter alia:

- The CEO has designated a suitably qualified employee as the CFO.
- The CEO and CFO have systems in place to keep proper accounts and financial records generally, a system for promptly preparing and auditing the annual financial statements, an assets register, and a system for the timely preparation of its annual report.
- The CEO and CFO have effective systems in place to receive, record, implement and monitor directions issued by the relevant Minister.
- An audit committee is in place.
- The audit committee has approved an internal audit charter.
- The risk management program includes a financial risk management program.
- The finance delegations meet the requirements of legislation.
- The CEO and CFO have systems in place to receive and respond promptly to requests for financial and other information from the relevant Minister.

Risk Management and Compliance

The health service Board must ensure that the health service also complies with mandatory risk

management requirements set out in the relevant mandatory risk management regimes.

This includes (inter alia) ensuring that health service:

(a) has an Enterprise Risk Management Framework developed in accordance with *ISO 31000:2009 Risk management—Principles and guidelines*[3]; and
(b) arranges all its insurance with the relevant medical indemnity insurance authority.

Other Legal Obligations

The Board ensures that the health service complies with all relevant legislation, including:

- Legislation relating to financial management and reporting obligations.
- Legislation relating to the administration of employee and patient information.
- Legislation relating to accountability and transparency requirements.
- Legislation relating to the safety and rights of mental health patients, such as the complaints.
- Legislation to improve the safety and protect the rights of employees.

The Board receives reporting on legislative compliance on an annual basis via the Audit Committee.

Health Service Board

The role and duties of the health service Board include strategy, governance and risk management.

The health service Board sets the strategic direction of the health service and monitors that health service is meeting its objectives and performance targets outlined in its Strategic Plan.

The health service Board has established this governance framework and monitors compliance

---

[3] https://www.iso.org/standard/43170.html.

with the framework. This framework covers the clinical work of the organisation, as well as the corporate and financial aspects of its operation.

The Board also ensures that risk management is integrated into health service's systems and reviews the effectiveness of operational risk management, compliance and reporting systems.

Board Functions

The Board must perform its functions and exercise its powers subject to any lawful direction given by the Minister and in accordance with the provisions of the relevant legislation. Additionally, the Board is responsible for the oversight of the implementation of government policy and guidelines issued from time to time from the Department of Health and other government agencies.

In brief, the role of the Board is to provide strategic direction for health service and effective oversight of management.

The functions of the Board are to:

- develop statements of priorities and strategic plans for the operation of health service and to monitor compliance with those statements and plans;
- develop financial and business plans, strategies and budgets to ensure the accountable and efficient provision of health services by the public health service and the long term financial viability of the public health service;
- establish and maintain effective systems to ensure that the health services provided meet the needs of the communities served by health service and that the views of users and providers of health services are taken into account;
- monitor the performance of health service to ensure that:
  - health service operates within its budget;
  - its audit and accounting systems accurately reflect the financial position and viability of health service;
  - health service adheres to its financial and business plans, strategic plans and statements of priorities;

- effective and accountable risk management systems are in place;
- effective and accountable systems are in place to monitor and improve the quality and effectiveness of health services provided by health service;
- any problems identified with the quality or effectiveness of the health services provided are addressed in a timely manner;
- health service continuously strives to improve the quality of the health services it provides and to foster innovation;
- Board sub-committees are established and operate effectively;
- appoint a chief executive officer of health service and to determine, subject to the government approval, his or her remuneration and the terms and conditions of appointment;
- monitor the performance of the chief executive officer of health service, each financial year, having regard to the objectives, priorities and key performance;
- establish the organisational structure, including the management structure, of health service;
- develop arrangements with other relevant agencies and service providers to enable effective and efficient service delivery and continuity of care;
- ensure that the relevant Minister and bureaucrat are advised about significant board decisions and are informed in a timely manner of any issues of public concern or risks that affect or may affect health service;
- establish a Finance Committee, an Audit Committee and a Quality Committee;
- facilitate health research and education;
- adopt a code of conduct for staff of health service;
- provide appropriate training for directors;
- any other functions conferred on the board by or under the relevant legislation;
- each year ensure that the Chief Executive Officer convenes an annual meeting during which the Board submits the report of operations and financial statements;

- appoint at least one community advisory committee and ensure that the persons appointed to the community advisory committee are persons who are able to represent the views of the communities served by health service;
- appoint a primary care and population health advisory committee and ensure that the persons appointed to the committee have the knowledge and expertise;
- include in its report of operations, a report on the activities of its advisory committees.

Board Obligations

Pursuant to its obligations set out in the relevant legislation, in performing its functions and exercising its powers, the health service Board must have regard to:

- the needs and views of patients and other users of the health services that health service provides and the community that health service serves;
- the need to ensure that health service uses its resources in an effective and efficient manner; and
- the need to ensure that resources of the public health sector generally are used effectively and efficiently.

Board Membership

The composition of the health services Board is usually set out in the relevant legislation.

The Board should include at least one person who is able to reflect the perspectives of users of health service and that women and men are adequately represented.

It is an expectation that Board members (inter alia):

- undertake identified and agreed training and development in order to fully discharge their responsibilities;
- bring to the attention of the Board chair any actual or perceived conflict of interest or potential conflict of interest;

- attend, at a minimum, 75% of Board meetings and any committee meeting they may be involved in during the year.

Board Chair

One of the directors must be appointed according to the relevant legislation to be the chairperson of the Board.

The position of Board chair is important because she or he is the major point of contact between the Chief Executive Officer and the Board, leads the Board and develops its members as an effective team. The chair has a particular role to play in relation to effective Board operation. This includes effective, efficient and constructive chairing of meetings and managing the evaluation of the CEO and Board. The Board chair is responsible for ensuring a Board evaluation, chair and individual director evaluations occur annually with an externally facilitated review at least every 3 years.

Board Selection

Board composition is important for board effectiveness. Appointments to the Board are usually made in consultation with the Board Chair. To maximise the Board's capacity for effective governance the right mix of skills, expertise and personal attributes are required. It is also important to achieve a balance between new members and ideas and corporate memory. The Board Chair and Directors, through the Board self-evaluation process, determine a view on the most effective composition for the Board, including skills mix and gaps, and provide advice on this to the Minister, if required.

Board Member Resignation and Removal

A director of the Board may resign in writing, signed by that person, and the appropriate body or individual as outlined in the relevant legislation may remove a director from office, if it is satisfied that the person:

- is physically or mentally unable to fulfil the role of director; or
- has been convicted of an offence, the commission of which, in the opinion of the Minister, makes the person unsuitable to be a director; or
- has been absent, without leave of the Board of directors, from all meetings of the Board of directors held during a period of 6 months; or
- is an insolvent under administration.

Board Committees

The Board delegates some aspects of its work to its committees. The committees are able to carry out a more detailed analysis of certain issues and make recommendations for the Board to consider. The Board remains accountable for all decisions.

Health service's Board committees are each established with:

- clear terms of reference;
- procedures for agendas, minutes and reporting to the Board; and
- appropriate membership.

On discharging their obligations, all committee members will ensure they take into consideration the health, safety and welfare of persons at health service in all decision making, including the promotion of a zero harm culture within the health service.

The Health service should establish the following committees:

- Audit Committee
- Quality Committee
- Remuneration Committee
- Finance Committee
- Consumer Advisory Committee
- Primary Care and Population Health Advisory Committee

Audit Committee

The Audit Committee is a Committee of the Board. The purpose of the Audit Committee is to assist health service and its Board by providing assurance in the key areas of statutory financial statements, internal control, legislative compliance and oversight of the activities of risk management, internal and external audit.

The role of the Audit Committee is as follows:

(a) independently review and assess the effectiveness of the health service's systems and controls for financial management, performance and sustainability, including risk management;
(b) oversee the internal audit function, including to:
    1. review and approve the internal audit charter;
    2. review and approve the strategic internal audit plan;
    3. review and approve the annual audit work program;
    4. review the effectiveness and efficiency of the function;
    5. advise the agency on the appointment and performance of the internal auditors; and
    6. meet privately with internal auditors if necessary;
(c) review annual financial statements and make a recommendation to the health service Board as to whether to authorise the statements;
(d) review information in the report of operations on financial management, performance and sustainability;
(e) review and monitor compliance with the relevant financial legislation, and advise the health service Board on the level of compliance attained;
(f) review and monitor remedial actions taken to address compliance deficiencies;
(g) maintain effective communication with external auditors, including by:
    1. understanding the external audit strategy and internal audit activities;

2. considering the external auditor's views on any issues, including accounting issues that may impact on the financial statements, financial management compliance issues and other relevant risks impacting the health service's finances;
3. considering external audit outcomes, including financial and performance audits;
4. providing a standing invitation to the external auditor to attend Audit Committee meetings; and
5. meeting privately at least once each year to ensure frank and open communication;

(h) consider recommendations made by internal and external auditors relating to or impacting on financial management, performance and sustainability and the actions to be taken by the health service to resolve issues raised; and
(i) regularly review implementation of actions in response to internal or external audits, including remedial actions to mitigate future instances of non-compliance.

The Audit Committee must be independent with:

(j) at least three members who are non-executive directors of the health service Board;
(k) an independent member as Chair (this must not be the Chair of the Board);
(l) self-assess its performance annually and report this assessment to the health service Board; and
(m) not include the following persons as members:
(n) the Chief Executive;
(o) Chief Financial Officer; or
(p) the internal auditors.

Quality Committee

The Quality Committee is a Committee of the Board of Directors. The purpose of the Quality Committee is to support the Board's function of providing strategic leadership in relation to the clinical governance of quality and safety at health service. It serves to ensure on behalf of the Board of Directors of health service, that the following broad objectives are fulfilled:

• Effective and accountable systems are in place to monitor and improve the quality and effectiveness of all health services provided by health service.
• Any problems identified with the quality or effectiveness of the health services provided are addressed in a timely manner.
• The health service continuously strives to improve the quality of all the health services it provides and to foster innovation.

Remuneration Committee

The principal role of the health service Remuneration Committee is to advise the Board of Directors on matters relating to the organisation's remuneration policies and practices.

In addition, the health service Remuneration Committee will provide oversight with respect to succession planning for the Chief Executive and senior executive positions.

Within the parameters established by the Board, the Remuneration Committee is responsible for:

• Developing and reviewing the organisation's executive remuneration policy and practices and ensuring that the strategies and performance of health service are taken into account.
• Advising the Board on "best practice" trends and practices in employment conditions and employee remuneration, including the changing legal requirements on executive and senior management remuneration.
• Recommending remuneration movements for the Chief Executive to the Board and for approving remuneration movements for senior executives and senior managers.

Finance Committee

The Finance Committee is a Committee of the Board of Directors. The purpose of the Finance

Committee is to advise the Board of Directors on financial matters impacting health service and to establish and maintain effective financial governance, including:

(a) an appropriate internal management structure and oversight arrangements for planning, managing and overseeing the financial operations, risks and opportunities of their health service to achieve performance and compliance;
(b) appropriate levels of resourcing and capability (including succession planning) to deliver health service's financial management, performance and sustainability obligations;
(c) clear roles, responsibilities, accountabilities and delegations that are documented and communicated;
(d) the development and implementation of policies and procedures to support the internal control system, in a way that is consistent with, and appropriate for, the sound financial management of health service's business operations;
(e) the effective management and oversight of health service's financial management activities that are undertaken externally, including shared services arrangements and outsourcing to private sector providers;
(f) effective relationships between stakeholders, committees of the Board and management;
(g) cooperation with external parties, including other Agencies, to achieve common objectives; and
(h) consideration of the effect of compliance burdens when developing and imposing requirements.

Specifically, the Finance Committee will review, monitor and report on the following:

• Financial strategy and direction;
• Financial performance and reporting;
• Financial risks;
• Capital planning, major projects, major tenders and business cases;
• Investments and cash flow;
• Balance sheet position; and
• Fundraising activities.
• Other matters specifically delegated to it by the Board.

Community Advisory Committee

The Community Advisory Committee is an advisory committee established by the Board of Directors. The Board must ensure that:

(a) persons appointed to the Community Advisory Committee are persons who are able to represent the view of the communities served by health service and
(b) In appointing persons to the Community Advisory Committee, preference is given to a person who is not a registered health practitioner, nor a person who is not currently or not recently been employed or engaged in the provision of health services.

The role of the Community Advisory Committee is to:

• Identify and advise the health service Board of Directors on priority areas and issues requiring a consumer, carer and/or community perspective.
• Advocate on behalf of consumers, carers and the community, including promoting greater attention and sensitivity to the needs of diverse, disadvantaged, isolated and marginalised consumers and communities.
• Provide direction on the development of a strategic Community Participation Plan for approval by the health service Board of Directors and monitor its implementation and effectiveness, including overseeing the preparation of an annual report to the Department of Health on progress against the Community Participation Plan.
• Provide direction and advice on the implementation of the accreditation standards relevant to consumers and patient experience, and monitor implementation and evaluation across health service.

- Participate in the health service strategic planning process and provide ongoing monitoring and input into the strategic priorities.
- Facilitate two-way communication between consumer, carer and community groups and health service.
- Participate in monitoring Quality and Safety measurements and Patient Centred Care key performance indicators for quality improvement.
- Assist in identifying development and training needs in relation to consumer, carer and community participation and make recommendation to the health service Board of Directors on how to meet these needs.

In undertaking these responsibilities, the Community Advisory Committee can seek information and briefings on health service core activities and programs.

Board Effectiveness and Evaluation

The Board evaluates its own performance annually, and undertakes an externally facilitated review at least every 3 years in order to identify areas of improvement and to provide development for the Directors' and the Board.

The Board Committees review their performance annually and provide recommendations to the Board of any actions that should be taken to improve the Committee's performance. Each Board Committee reviews its Charter annually.

Delegations to the Health Service Executive

The Board has delegated powers to the CEO and Executive. The delegations of authority provide a list of functions that have been delegated by the Board. The delegation manual includes a description of the delegated power and any conditions limiting the exercise of those powers (including financial limits).

The delegations are reviewed annually by the Finance Committee and approved by the Board.

Directors' Ethical and Legal Obligations

Code of Conduct

The public health service directors' are subject to the Directors' code of conduct. The code of conduct expresses the public sector values in terms that are most relevant to the special role and duties of Directors. The Directors' code of conduct is based on the same set of values (the public sector values) that apply to all public officials, including employees.

A health service director must:

- Act with *honesty and integrity*. Be open and transparent in their dealings; use power responsibly; not place oneself in a position of conflict of interest; strive to earn and sustain public trust of a high level.
- Act in *good faith in the best interests of health service*. Demonstrate accountability for their actions; accept responsibility for their decisions; not engage in activities that may bring themselves or health service into disrepute.
- Act *fairly and impartially*. Avoid bias, discrimination, caprice or self-interest; demonstrate respect for others by acting in a professional and courteous manner.
- *Use information appropriately.* Ensure information gained as a director is only applied to proper purposes and is kept confidential.
- *Use their position appropriately.* Not use their position as a director to seek an undue advantage for oneself, family members or associates, or to cause detriment to health service; decline gifts or favours that may cast doubt on their ability to apply independent judgment as a health service Board member.
- Act in a *financially responsible* manner. Understand financial reports, audit reports and other financial material that comes before the health service Board; actively inquire into this material.
- Exercise *due care, diligence and skill.* Ascertain all relevant information; make

reasonable enquiries; understand the financial, strategic and other implications of decisions.

- *Comply with the establishing legislation* for the health service.
- Demonstrate *leadership and stewardship.* Promote and support the application of the Victorian public sector values; act in accordance with the Directors' Code.

Conflicts of Interest

The Directors' code of conduct requires Directors to act with honesty and integrity and to act in the best interests of health service. This means avoiding placing themselves in a position of conflict of interest. Obligations in relation to conflicts of interests are further articulated in the health service's Conflict of Interest Policies.

Duties of Directors

Health service Directors must act honestly, in good faith in the best interests of health service, with integrity, in a financially responsible manner, with a reasonable degree of care, diligence and skill, and in compliance with relevant legislation.

Health service Directors must not give to any other person, directly or indirectly, any information acquired through being a director (apart from when carrying out functions authorised, permitted or required under an Act).

Health service Directors must not improperly use his or her position, or any information acquired through that position, to gain a personal advantage, or for the advantage of another person, or to cause detriment to health service.

Declaration of Private Interests

Health service Directors' are required to complete an updated Declaration of Private Interests on an annual basis. Any perceived or actual conflict of interest which is declared by a director is to be managed in accordance with the health service Conflict of Interest Policy.

Health Service's Executive Committee

The health service's Executive Committee is responsible for the day to day running of health service, in accordance with the law, the decisions of the Board and government policies.

Chief Executive Officer

The Board appoints the Chief Executive Officer (CEO) of health service and determines, subject to the Secretary's approval, the CEO's remuneration and the terms and conditions of his or her appointment.

The CEO is subject to the direction of the Board in controlling and managing health service. The functions of the CEO are:

- to prepare material for consideration by the Board, including the Strategic Plan;
- to ensure that health service uses its resources effectively and efficiently;
- to implement service development and planning; and
- any other functions as specified by the Board.

The role of the CEO is to:

- manage the effective and efficient operations of health service in accordance with the strategy, business plans and policies of the Board;
- implement Board decisions;
- ensure health service's organisational functions are effective, including financial management, human resource management, asset management and reporting;
- maintain effective communication and cooperation with stakeholders in collaboration with the Chair of the Board;
- oversee the employment and management of staff;
- provide advice and information to the Board on any material issues concerning strategy, finance, reporting obligations and significant events that require the Board to notify the Minister and Department of Health;

- prepare health service's Annual Report;
- liaise with the Department of Health; and
- represent health service to external parties as an official spokesperson for health service, in consultation with the Chair of the Board.

The CEO is usually the accountable officer for health service the relevant legislation. As the accountable officer, the CEO must:

- designate an employee as the CFO, and designate other staff who receive money and make payments;
- ensure that proper accounts and records are kept;
- provide the Minister for Health or the Minister for Finance any financial information they request;
- prepare financial statements and report of operations;
- complete the annual Financial Management Compliance Framework as soon as possible after the end of each financial year;
- write off debts, losses or deficiency in health service accounts in accordance with the regulations; and
- organise investigations into the loss, deficiency or destruction of public money or property that may have been caused by a serving or former office of health service and decides whether to try to recover funds from that officer.

Chief Financial Officer (CFO)

The CFO is responsible for health service's financial accounting and financial reporting, the effectiveness of health service's audit arrangements and the efficient and effective use of resources. The CFO is responsible to the CEO for ensuring that proper accounting records and systems and other records are maintained in accordance with the relevant regulations.

The CFO may provide the Board with advice on:

- the financial statements;
- compliance with legislation;

- the internal control systems to avoid fraud and misappropriation;
- liaison with external auditors;
- the audit process;
- action taken on audit reports; and
- managing financial risk.

External Regulatory and Monitoring

The health service is subject to regulation and oversight from a number of external bodies.

The Government

The Department of Health and government agencies have a number of key clinical governance responsibilities including:

- setting expectations and requirements regarding health service accountability for quality and safety and continuous improvement;
- ensuring health services have the necessary data to fulfil their responsibilities, including benchmarked and trend data;
- providing leadership, support and direction to ensure safe, high-quality healthcare can be provided;
- ensuring board members have the required skills and knowledge to fulfil their responsibilities;
- proactively identifying and responding decisively to emerging clinical quality and safety trends;
- effectively monitoring the implementation and performance of clinical governance systems, ensuring the early identification of risks and flags; and
- monitoring clinical governance implementation and performance by continually reviewing key quality and safety indicators.

Accreditation of the Health Service

Accreditation is part of the regulatory framework that informs government and the community that systems are present in health services to protect the public from harm and improve the quality of health service provision.

The health service maintains accreditation through an independent, external accreditation body. The accreditation process is a formal process of external review based on a series of standards of care and processes. Health services are all required to be accredited by certain specified bodies. The health service is also accredited and monitored against the relevant mental health and aged care accreditation bodies as relevant.

Health Service Governance Framework Checklist

The following table is a summary of the actions taken by the health service Board to ensure it acts in accordance with its eight governance principles.

Principle		Action
Establish robust governance and oversight frameworks	☑	Members of the board, the Chief Executive and the senior management of health service are aware of the governance requirements for health service as set out in the health service Governance Framework
	☑	The governance structures required by the health service Board Charter, statutory instruments and government policy are established to provide effective oversight of clinical and corporate responsibilities
	☑	Accountabilities for health service delivery are clearly established at health service
	☑	The authorities reserved for the Monash health Board and those delegated to management are clearly documented and reviewed annually
	☑	The Board—OH&S—Code of Conduct
	☑	The Board and chief executive can demonstrate compliance with the eight corporate governance standards approved by the Board
Effective and accountable systems are in place to monitor and improve the quality of the health services provided	☑	The Board ensures that effective safety and quality systems and robust organisational structures are in place, that their performance is monitored and that health service responds appropriately to safety and quality problems
	☑	The health service Board are responsible and accountable for ensuring the systems and processes are in place to support clinicians in providing safe, high-quality care, and in ensuring clinicians participate in governance activities in accordance with the Safer Care Victoria Clinical Governance Framework
	☑	The responsibility for designing and implementing systems and monitoring the effectiveness of clinical care is appropriately delegated to managers and health care professionals with specific expertise. Clinicians and clinical teams are responsible and accountable for the safety and quality of care they provide
	☑	The Board ensures it receives systematic reports across the range of quality and safety assurance activities
	☑	The Board ensures that health service participates in regular assessments to maintain accreditation to ensure that it meets quality and safety standards in service delivery
Set the strategic direction for the organisation and its services	☑	The strategic plan is developed in accordance with Ministerial guidelines
	☑	Agree an annual Statement of Priorities with the Minister
	☑	Prepare an annual quality account report
	☑	Quarterly reporting under the Victorian Health Services Performance Monitoring Framework
	☑	Monitoring service delivery performance
	☑	Foster research and education by ensuring key partnerships are in place
	☑	Ensure progress towards integrated care by ensuring key partnerships
Monitor financial and service delivery performance	☑	Approve financial and operating plans and budges to ensure the accountable and efficient provision of health services and the viability of health service
	☑	Monitor financial performance monthly
	☑	Reviewing the capital plan
	☑	Approving the annual financial statements
	☑	Reviewing and approving investment strategies in accordance with government policy

Principle		Action
Maintain high standards of professional and ethical conduct	☑	The Board complies with the Director's Code of Conduct issued by the Public Sector Standards Commissioner
	☑	Health service Board members disclose any conflicts of interest and declare personal interests in accordance with government policy
	☑	The Board reviews and approves the health service Code of Conduct and ensures that its obligations are enforced
	☑	A Fraud and Corruption Policy is in place
	☑	A Gifts and Benefits Policy is in place and monitored
	☑	All instances of improper conduct are managed properly and reported externally where relevant
Involve stakeholders in decisions that affect them	☑	Information is published on the internet, including quality of care reports, annual reports and privacy information
	☑	An effective complaints management process is in place.
	☑	Health service has a Community Participation Plan which is embedded in the health service Strategic Plan
	☑	Ensure that health service has programs demonstrating a commitment to diversity
	☑	Aboriginal Liaison
	☑	health service is responsive to statutory agencies such as the Coroner, IBAC, Mental Health Complaints Commissioner, Health Care Complaints Commissioner and the Ombudsman
Establish sound audit and risk management practices	☑	A compliance program is in place to ensure the legal and policy obligations of health service are identified, understood and managed
	☑	Health service's Enterprise Risk Management Framework has been developed in accordance with ISO 31000:2009 Risk management—Principles and guidelines
	☑	Health service complies with the Victorian Government Risk Framework, including the requirement to arrange for its insurance with the VMIA
	☑	An internal audit function is in place and accountable to the Board
	☑	The Board regularly reviews health service's governance framework including policies and procedures
	☑	The Board approves and regularly reviews the Delegations of Authority
	☑	The Audit Committee reviews management controls and strategies associated with high and medium risks
	☑	The Board ensures that the Internal Auditors have access to the health service Board via the Audit committee and has sufficient information to perform its function
Ensure key partnerships to develop integrated care, research and education	☑	The health service Translation Precinct (MHTP) brings the research, education and clinical expertise of health service, Monash University and the Hudson Institute of Medical Research and health service together

Prasad Godbole and Derek Burke

Case Study

The Mid Staffs 'scandal' [1] arose from concerns raised by the public into the treatment of patients at the Mid Staffordshire Hospitals NHS Foundation Trust. These concerns were raised over a number of years and culminated in the Francis report in 2013 (https://www.health.org.uk/about-the-francis-inquiry). As part of the Francis report there were several key points noted:

1. Patients were not put first and care was not patient centred
2. Staffing was reduced and skill mix diluted to cut costs
3. Board meetings were held in private with lack of communication that led to an element of mistrust.
4. There was significant disconnect between management and frontline staff who felt disengaged
5. Reporting of untoward incidents or concerns was not encouraged and even when concerns by staff were raised, these were largely ignored
6. The organisational culture did not promote safety
7. Staff morale was low and there were instances of bullying against staff who voiced concerns
8. The main focus of the hospital was target driven priorities rather than patient safety
9. There was lack of honesty and transparency (candour) when things went wrong
10. There was a sense of denial at senior management level that anything was wrong as these shortcomings were felt to be similar to other Trusts in the region and hence 'they were no different'

As a result of this inquiry, several key recommendations (https://www.gov.uk/government/news/francis-report-on-mid-staffs-government-accepts-recommendations) were made and implemented throughout the NHS

1. A common culture has been proposed throughout the NHS
2. The report placed emphasis on the creation of a safety culture
3. An organisation should have shared values between management and frontline staff
4. The NHS must have a strong consistent leadership to motivate staff

P. Godbole (✉)
Department of Paediatric Surgery, Sheffield Children's NHS Foundation Trust, Sheffield, UK
e-mail: Prasad.Godbole@sch.nhs.uk

D. Burke
Department of Emergency Medicine, Sheffield Children's NHS Foundation Trust, Sheffield, UK
e-mail: Derek.Burke@sch.nhs.uk

© Springer Nature Switzerland AG 2019
D. Burke et al. (eds.), *Hospital Transformation*, https://doi.org/10.1007/978-3-030-15448-6_11

5. Everyone employed by the NHS should have a questioning attitude, a rigorous approach and good communication skills.

While patient safety is paramount and should always be the foremost priority in any healthcare service, why do hospitals still find themselves not performing to standards either from the patient perspective or not being able to balance the books? Let us look at the key requirements of what can make a hospital successful

Organisational Level

1. Leadership: a lot has been written about leadership in healthcare organisations and what constitutes a good leader. However leadership in the context of transformation can be a challenging [2]. A leader has to be brave and bold and committed to the vision and values of the organisation. The leader should have a clear vision about the short medium and longer term endpoints for the organisation (where do we want to be) and be able to communicate this vision effectively to all staff members, particularly to the frontline staff. The leader should be visible to staff and lead by his/her own behaviour. At the same time the leader should be firm and be able to stand their ground when they firmly believe a particular strategic direction is not right for the organisation.

2. Communication and Engagement: engagement between management and frontline staff is key for the success of any transformation project [3]. This engagement should be more a 'listening' and not a 'telling' exercise. Far too often this engagement of frontline staff is only paid lip service in real life. Visibility of the management team is also of significant importance [4]. In many organisations frontline staff report that they have no idea who the management team is apart from the notion that they sit in the 'executive corridor '. This lack of engagement and open lines of communication leads to a culture of them against us in relation to transformation. Engagement has to be truly collaborative and not simply a gesture.

3. Transparency: Staff have a right to know how their organisation is performing, when things go wrong and what is being done to manage errors and prevent future errors occurring. It is essential that staff buy in to the transformational vision and the rationale for the transformational change for it to succeed.

4. Organisational culture: Following the Francis report, many organisations have redefined their organisational culture. These new cultures are centred around organisational honesty and a duty of candour when things have gone wrong, encouraging incident reporting and most importantly putting patients first and at the heart of everything the organisation does.

5. Performance management and accountability framework: many organisations have an organisational structure which includes a board and executive management team. The non executive directors should be in a position to challenge the executive team and in turn the executive team should be able to performance manage those who are not performing adequately. However it is still common in many organisations to find executive management teams who do not challenge performance or poor outcomes. In government funded health systems the executives may be restricted in the actions they can take in relation to performance management [5].

6. Workforce: it is essential that organisations have the right number and skill mix of workforce to do the job. Frontline workforce both clinical and non clinical should have the relevant expertise and experience to provide high quality care. Support for the workforce in terms of funding for continuing professional development should be a given. Lack of provision of such funding can have the effect of demoralising the workforce and lead to deskilling and risks to patient safety.

7. Engaging with external stakeholders: organisations cannot operate in isolation but have to operate as part of the overall healthcare system in which they operate. This may include working with stakeholders such as community based teams, school based teams for

children, mental health and social care teams. Working as a collaborative group can assist in driving change across the spectrum of health and social care.

Delivery of Patient Care

1. Patient focused: any healthcare service provider should have the patient at the heart of everything they do. Treatment and care should be provided based on what individuals in the organisation would expect if they or their families were patients themselves. The overall patient experience should be a positive one.
2. Outcomes oriented: Benchmarking against national and international standards for outcomes as well as devising a list of quality indicators for the organisation is important as it allows an organisation to know whether it is doing a good job in the delivery of its service.
3. Data insights: the amount of data that an organisation can generate is significant: activity data and performance data by speciality and individual clinician, outcomes data, peer review data, financial data, quality data and audit data. However this data is of little use if it has not been properly analysed to produce information which allows executives and non-executives to make judgements about the absolute and relative performance of the organisation.
4. Root cause analysis: where things go wrong, there needs to be a team of individuals skilled in undertaking a root cause analysis of the problem. To ensure that the true root of the error is addressed. Currently many organisations will only undertake a RCA for patient related safety incidents that cross a trigger risk threshold rather than as a routine for failure in other areas.

Financial

1. Cost effective: for any service to be viable, it has to be cost effective and provide value for money. With emerging new technologies and treatments, there has to be good evidence that they provide safe, cost effective interventions and outcomes.

2. Reduce waste (LEAN) (https://www.leanproduction.com/intro-to-lean.html): in the US, it is reported that about 30% of national healthcare expenditure does not make any difference to or improve people's lives [6]. Reduction in waste and the use of LEAN or similar methodologies in every process can yield significant savings that can be reinvested in other key priorities.
3. Financial priorities: every organisation will have key financial priorities for delivery of healthcare services. Funding for patient safety and quality improvements are important but compete for funding with other priorities such as IT systems and newer technologies such as AI as well as priorities for workforce to deliver. Balancing these competing priorities is challenging particularly when there is no objective criteria for deriving the optimum allocation to each area. For example increasing the workforce in the emergency department rather than transforming working practices may reduce funding allocation for the housekeeping department which may in turn lead to lower levels of cleanliness, increased risk of hospital acquired infection and poor patient experience.

So What Is Transformation?

The term transformation is often used, even at senior management level, to reflect minor service changes or service improvements. Increasing the number of patients operated on in the operating rooms is not a transformation but should be a part of normal operational efficiency. However a whole scale change in working practices including a radical shift in the number of hours or days worked by OR staff including clinicians and revised workforce planning to maximise the efficiency could be termed a transformational change. It is important to differentiate between a radical change and merely 'tinkering' around the edges. While the steps towards achieving a successful transformation are mainly focused on the senior management team, it is essential for all members of staff to be aware of and engaged in the process. Transformation without staff engagement is doomed to fail. Transformation is a radical and irreversible change in the way a service is delivered, the way staff work and behave, how the patients are engaged with a view to a sustained and measurable improvement in patient focused service delivery and outcomes. It is dynamic iterative process which will span many years and is a continual cycle of identify, transform, embed and review.

Steps to a Successful Transformation and How Is It Done?

In any transformational change process, it is important to identify the focus for the transformation. In the case of healthcare organisations these may be divided into three intertwined broad interdependencies.

1. Finance: is necessary to deliver the activity required to generate the revenue and operational capital for the hospital. Finance is also required to deliver the quality and safety agenda of the hospital
2. Performance: the predicted activity that has been budgeted for has to be delivered. Failure to deliver this will reduce revenue and operational capital.
3. Quality and safety: patients nowadays have greater expectations from their healthcare providers than ever before and this trend is likely to continue. High quality care delivered with patient collaboration (shared care model) with good outcomes and good patient experience provides the potential of increased referrals (patient choice), greater market share for the organisation and increased revenue. Regulators also play a role in providing insight into areas required for improvement within hospitals.

The leadership team need to analyse the data available for all the above, review the interrelation-

ships between them in terms of causal and temporal linkage and identify areas for transformation.

Kotters 8 step transformation model [7] can be utilised and is outlined below:

1. Create a sense of urgency: the leadership team need to start talking to every member of staff about the need for transformation and the urgency of this transformation. Staff need to understand the organisational position in the marketplace and its strengths, weaknesses, opportunities and threats. The strategic short medium and long term vision needs to be communicated effectively and widely. This engagement needs to be by the leadership team (executive management) and not a delegated responsibility to the middle/junior management teams to the exclusion of senior managers. Getting the staff talking about the change process will allow negative thinkers and late adopters to have a chance to discuss this and get engaged in the conversations. According to Dr Kotter at least 75% of the workforce needs to be engaged and have a buy in for a successful transformation
2. Establish a transformation group: this is key to the success of a transformation project. Enthusiastic leaders need to be signed up to take on the roles within the transformation group. This is where the hierarchy of the management structure ends. The classical hierarchy of executive board of directors, middle managers and frontline staff should not be slavishly adhered to. Cooperation of clinicians and allied healthcare staff and non clinical staff as key stakeholders should be sought. It is the frontline staff who have the expertise and know how to able to solve problems or provide clinical input into different ways of achieving the goals of transformation. Very often decisions are made at executive board level with minimal representation from the clinical teams which therefore destined the transformation to fail. Utilising clinical champions and making them feel worth their role in

the transformation project will enable these clinicians to move the project forward. Currently in many organisations the role of middle managers is not well described apart from deputising or assisting senior managers in various meetings about transformation projects.

3. Define the end goal: the leadership team need to be able to clearly and concisely describe the end point of the transformation project and how it envisages getting to that end point. Many organisations do know the end point but are unable to identify how the change process will be implemented. This leads to a disjointed and quite often segmented way of thinking which is neither coherent or rational.

4. Share the end goal: once the end point is identified, this must be shared with all staff members through face to face meetings. Communications by email or various other means can lead to uncertainty and can raise more questions than are answered. Visibility of the leadership team is important when sharing the vision and the end goal.

5. Encourage participation and remove obstacles to participation: transformation is a dynamic process and does not happen overnight. There is always resistance to change and active discussion and collaborative efforts goes a long way in overcoming the resistance to change. There may be many hurdles and obstacles encountered in encouraging individuals to participate and any major hurdles should be removed. This may be giving clinicians time away from their clinical activity to participate in the transformational change rather than expecting them to do this as an added 'extra' to their role.

6. Share and celebrate short term gains: transformation gains should target 'low hanging fruit' and gains that are achievable in the short term without unnecessary expense. There is nothing more rewarding then for teams to be congratulated for achieving their short term goal and this motivates the team to persevere with the transformation.

7. Persist in driving change: failure to achieve short term gains can lead to a demoralising effect on the teams involved. However positive reinforcement and regular encouragement and feedback will enable teams to continue to drive change and be proud of their accomplishments.

8. Connect change to company culture: any transformational change has to be linked to the organisational culture. In case of healthcare organisations, the organisational culture should be one that is patient focused in every aspect with a culture of transparency and honesty. The organisation should be committed to continual improvement and any changes should be in this context rather than the unfortunate issue of financial savings that often forms the basis of transformational change.

Case Study 2: Putting It into Practice

A hospital in the south of England was put into special measures by the regulatory bodies—the CQC [8] and MONITOR [9] due to concerns over patient safety and quality of care. This was as reported by the BBC precipitated by the death of a 10 year old girl [10]. The following Table 11.1 demonstrates how the transformation of the hospital from being in 'special measures' to achieving a 'good' status was achieved.

Conclusion

Transformational change in a hospital setting is challenging. Most transformational changes fail due to lack of leadership, vision, engagement and communication. A whole team approach is necessary rather than an us (management) and them (clinicians) approach. Multiple stakeholders outside the normal hierarchy should be engaged in the process. Regular feedback and incentivising short term gains assists in a continual transformation process to achieve the long term vision (Table 11.2).

Table 11.1 Hospital transformation case study

No	Corrective action	Commentary
1	Chairman, CEO, executive management team replaced	Poor Leadership was replaced with a team that had the leadership qualities to drive the change
2	Data analysed, Root causes found, problems identified, key priorities agreed	The team appointed and replaced managers with those who were able to undertake and provide a coherent explanation for the data. This allowed the team to agree priorities
3	Clinical engagement and visibility	A meeting was held every morning in the canteen where anyone was welcome to attend and voice their concerns. The meeting lasted 20 min and was lead by the CEO. Similar meetings were held across departments by executive team frequently allowing them to gain an understanding of the problems but also allowing collaboration with the frontline workers
4	Clinical champions appointed	Clinicians as leaders were involved and engaged in the process
5	Service improvements identified, processes changed	As part of the transformation process, several programs of work were identified and commenced leading to service improvements and better patient safety
6	Feedback to staff	Communication constantly maintained
7	Hospital taken out of special measures	Hospital achieved key regulatory requirements and standards of patient safety and quality
8	Hospital has significant financial deficit	The hospital had to invest in the turnaround process. This caused them to go into deficit. However they have a robust plan for financial recovery over 3 years. It is a common mistake for hospitals to have finance as their key priority in terms of balancing the books. Sensible and strategic investment is important as long as a strong plan for recovery is agreed

Table 11.2 Self assessment 'health' checklist for healthcare organisations

	Green (2 points)	Amber (1 point)	Red (0 Points)
Leadership			
Does the chairman and non-executive directors have a track record in delivery of healthcare transformation	Yes		No
Is the CEO experienced in leading a executive management team	More than 5 years	1–5 years	Less than 1 year
How many transformation projects have the executive management team led that have been successful and can be communicated to staff in the last 5 years	More than 5	1–5	None
What percentage of staff know the executive management team by face and their role	More than 75%	25–75%	Less than 25%
How many times a week do members of the management team do a walk around the hospital gaining insight into daily operations and challenges	Every day	2–4 times a week	Less than twice a week
How many times a week are open forums held and led by a member of the executive team	Every day	Every week	Less than monthly
How often are views of the workforce sought	Weekly	Monthly	Annually
What percentage of the workforce would agree that there is clear communication and engagement about the vision, strategy, rationale and implementation of a transformation program	More than 75%	25–75%	Less than 25%
What percentage of the staff are aware of the vision, values and organisational culture	More than 75%	25–75%	Less than 25%

Table 11.2 (continued)

	Green (2 points)	Amber (1 point)	Red (0 Points)
Do all managers have job descriptions and key performance indicators available for review at any time	Yes all have job descriptions and KPI	50–75% have job descriptions and KPI	Less than 50% have job descriptions and KPI
Is there evidence of performance management and remedial actions as a result	Documentary evidence for more than 75% of teams/managers	Documentary evidence 50–75%	Documentary evidence less than 50% of the time
Has there been any compulsory redundancies made from the hospital in the last 5 years due to poor performance	Yes		No
Workforce			
Are there enough clinicians for the activity to be delivered	Yes		No
Is there the correct skill mix of clinicians	Yes		No
Are clinical leaders identified and have they got a track record in transformation	Yes		No
Have clinicians been supported to develop skills as leaders	Yes		No
Are clinicians supported financially for CPD	Yes	Partially funded	No
What percentage of clinicians would state they are actively encouraged to engage in the hospital operations and change processes	More than 75%	50–75%	Less than 50%
What percentage of clinicians feel the hospital is too 'management heavy' or not fit for purpose	More than 75%	50–75%	Less than 50%
What is the incidence of long term sickness amongst clinicians	Less than 1%	1–3%	Greater than 3%
How many clinicians as a percentage of clinical workforce attend open forums if organised	Greater than 75%	50–75%	Less than 50%
What percentage of identified clinical leaders are in charge of transformation projects	Greater than 75%	50–75%	Less than 50%
Does the hospital have an adequate nurse establishment across all departments	Yes		No
Is the nursing skill mix appropriate	Yes		No
What percentage of nurses feel they are engaged in hospital transformation	Greater than 75%	50–75%	Less than 50%
Are nursing leaders identified and contribution to transformation documented	Yes		No
What is the sickness incidence amongst nursing staff	1–2%	3–5%	Greater than 5%
Are nurses supported for CPD financially	Yes		No
Non clinical workforce and allied healthcare workforce			
Are there adequate staff and skill mix	Yes		No
Are there staff able to undertake RCA and how many	Yes more than 5	Currently 3–5	No less than 3
How many data analysts form part of the workforce who can interrogate the data for answers	Yes more than 3	Currently 1–3	None
What is the overall staff sickness	1–2%	2–5%	Greater than 5%
Is the staff sickness increasing, same or decreasing over the last 5 years	Decreasing	Same	Increasing

(continued)

Table 11.2 (continued)

	Green (2 points)	Amber (1 point)	Red (0 Points)
Delivery of patient care			
Does the hospital have robust evidence to demonstrate evidence based care	Yes		No
Have the patient related safety incidents remained the same, decreased or increased over the last 5 years	Decreasing	Same	Increasing
How many complaints have been received and have they stayed the same, increased or decreased over the last 5 years	Decreasing	Same	Increasing
How many deaths have been avoidable and are all deaths reported and investigated	All	Some	None
How many serious incidents have been reported annually and have these increased, decreased or stayed the same over the last 5 years	Decreasing	Same	Increasing
What percentage of patients/families would recommend your hospital to relatives/friends	Greater than 98%	85–98%	Less than 85%
Has your hospital received a poor rating for any service by regulators	No	Don't know	Yes
What percentage of patients/families would describe the hospital as clean and pleasant	Greater than 98%	85–98%	Less than 85%
What percentage of staff, families and patients describe the catering facilities in the hospital as good	Greater than 98%	85–98%	Less than 85%
What percentage of patients per annum have contracted avoidable complications such as DVT, MRSA, pressure ulcer, venous ulcer, C. Difficile	None	Less than 1%	Greater than 1%
What percentage of patients and families surveyed would state they have met a member of the management team to ask their views of the service provided	Greater than 98%	85–98%	Less than 85%
Does the hospital publish outcome data by clinician on their website	Yes		No
Finance			
Is the hospital in surplus, break even or in deficit	Surplus	Break-even	Deficit
Is the hospital delivering on activity in terms of performance across all specialities	Yes	In some specialities	No
Is the hospital achieving any internal standards of performance and productivity	Yes	In some specialities	No
Is there a documented integrated root cause analysis identifying key factors for the financial position	Yes	Partial	No
Is there a documented investment and recovery plan that is robust	Yes		No
Is there any regulatory pressure on the hospital for financial stability	No		Yes
Are transformation and investment projects on hold due to financial considerations	No	Some plans are on hold	Yes, all plans are on hold
What percentage of the workforce feel finance is a key priority for the hospital as well as cost cutting	Less than 25%	25–75%	More than 75%

Table 11.2 (continued)

	Green (2 points)	Amber (1 point)	Red (0 Points)
Organisational			
Number of successful litigations over the last 5 years	Decreasing	No change	Increasing
Percentage of budget over the last 5 years on settling claims of all types	Decreasing	No change	Increasing
Staff retention over the last 5 years	More than 85%	More than 75%	Less than 75%

Note: maximum score = 114. 85% of maximum = good no changes needed, continue transformation, efficiency projects; 50–75% of maximum = needs remedial action; Less than 50% = needs urgent remedial intervention

References

1. Holmes D. Mid Staffordshire scandal highlights NHS cultural crisis. The Lancet. 2013;381(9866):521–2.
2. Walsh N. The leadership challenges of sustainability and transformation plans. London: The Kings Fund; 2016. Available at https://www.kingsfund.org.uk/blog/2016/04/leadership-challenges-stps.
3. Daneshgari P, Moore H. Organizational transformation through improved employee engagement – "How to use effective methodologies to improve business productivity and expand market share". Strategic HR Rev. 2016;15(2):57–64.
4. Kotter JP. Leading change: why transformation efforts fail. Harvard Business Review. 1995. Available at https://hbr.org/1995/05/leading-change-why-transformation-efforts-fail-2.
5. Lutwama GW, Roos JH, Dolamo BL. Assessing the implementation of performance management of health care workers in Uganda. BMC Health Serv Res. 2013;13:355.
6. Obama B. United States Health care reform: progress to date and next steps. JAMA. 2016;316(5):525–32.
7. Webster V, Webster M. Successful change management — Kotter's 8-Step Change Model. Available at https://www.leadershipthoughts.com/kotters-8-step-change-model/.
8. https://www.cqc.org.uk.
9. https://improvement.nhs.uk.
10. https://www.bbc.com/news/uk-england-essex-25309619.

Stephen Stericker and Dawn Lawson

Introduction

Much has been written about improvement and transformation in the NHS and is covered elsewhere in this book. The most significant challenge in the transformation process is ensuring that change or improvement is sustained over time, after the 'initiative' has ended. Often, when embarking on a transformation initiative, there can be little, if any, thought put into the sustainability of the transformation. Similarly, there is sometimes inadequate attention paid to the evaluation of the impact of the transformation.

In our experience of undertaking transformation and seeking to ensure that it is sustained, there are several key elements that must be considered from the outset. Our conclusion is that whether or not the transformation will be sustained must depend from the start on how you engage, construct implement and evaluate it, rather than being too pre-occupied with the subject of the transformation itself.

We will discuss the context for sustainability in NHS acute hospitals and describe guidance from various sources. We then move on to describe the importance of working in partnership with others, both internal and external to an organisation.

It is critical to recognise that any transformation sits within a wider system of constant change that will either enable sustainable change or present challenges to overcome. We hope this chapter provides some practical advice that can be contextualised to help you ensure the transformation outcomes that you work on are sustained.

The Context for Sustainability in NHS Acute Hospitals

Thinking about sustainability in acute hospitals means thinking about the local regional and national environment or context within which they are operating. In 2014, the NHS 5 Year Forward View [1] emphasised the need to get serious about prevention.

> The future health of millions of children, the sustainability of the NHS, and the economic prosperity all now depend on a radical upgrade in prevention and public health [1, p. 9]

The NHS 5 Year Forward View describes three improvement opportunities: a health gap, a quality gap, and a financial sustainability gap. In order to address these gaps, it explores opportunities to steer the 'triple integration' of primary and specialist hospital care, of physical and mental health services, and of health and social care. It is considered to be the role of the NHS and a well-functioning public health and social care sector to bring about any necessary changes.

S. Stericker, PhD (✉)
Care to Innovate, NHS and Social Care, York, UK
e-mail: stephen_stericker@sky.com

D. Lawson
Liverpool Health Partners, Liverpool, UK

© Springer Nature Switzerland AG 2019
D. Burke et al. (eds.), *Hospital Transformation*, https://doi.org/10.1007/978-3-030-15448-6_12

The Care Quality Commission published *The state of care in NHS acute hospitals: 2014–2016* [2]. The report identified demographic population changes leading to rising demand for services, coupled with economic pressures. The financial challenge was reported to be significant for all NHS providers, with a 2015/2016 deficit of £2.45 billion and 60% of all acute trusts forecasting a year-end deficit for 2016/2017.

Professor Mike Richards stated the following:

> The NHS stands on a burning platform—the model of acute care that worked well when the NHS was established is no longer capable of delivering the care that today's population needs. The need for change is clear, but finding the resources and energy to deliver change while simultaneously providing safe patient care can seem near impossible. [2, p. 4]

In 2017, the Next Steps on the NHS 5 Year Forward View supported the need for strategic partnerships to plan and integrate the commissioning and delivery of health and care services:

> We now want to accelerate this way of working to more of the country, through partnerships of care providers and commissioners in an area (Sustainability and Transformation Partnerships). Some areas are now ready to go further and more fully integrate their services and funding, and we will back them in doing so (Accountable Care Systems). Working together with patients and the public, NHS commissioners and providers, as well as local authorities and other providers of health and care services, they will gain new powers and freedoms to plan how best to provide care, while taking on new responsibilities for improving the health and wellbeing of the population they cover. [3, p. 5]

Ham et al. [4] published a report that reviewed proposals in 44 Sustainable Transformation Plans submitted to NHS England. Key messages for the acute hospital sector included planned reductions in the number of acute hospital beds, using existing services in the community more effectively to moderate demand for hospital care and reconfiguring hospitals.

NHS Improvement affirmed their commitment to support the implementation of priorities contained within the Next Steps on the NHS 5 Year Forward View. The NHS Improvement Business Plan 2017–2019 [5] reflected a focus on developing "a clinically, operationally and financially sustainable pattern of care and implementing strategic changes". The plan makes it clear that providers will be required to transform services by developing and adopting new care models and new models of accountable care. A key priority for NHS Improvement is to support those organisations seeking to become accountable care organisations (ACOs). It is expected that ACOs will manage an integrated budget for primary, community, mental health and acute care and be responsible for improving the health outcomes for a defined population.

The context for the wider public sector is also one of severe pressures, with Government funding for local authorities having fallen by an estimated 49.1% in real terms from 2010–2011 to 2017–2018. [6, p. 4]. Alongside reductions in funding, local authorities have experienced growth in demand for key services, as well as absorbing other cost pressures. It is therefore not surprising that acute NHS hospitals have experienced continuing delays in discharging patients into overstretched community and social care services.

To address the 'burning platform' of sustainable health and social care services, a consistent policy solution across the NHS and Local Government has seen guidance developed to encourage health and social care commissioners to work in more integrated ways. The Local Government Association and the NHS published *Integrated Commissioning for Better Outcomes: A Commissioning Framework* [7] to support local health and care economies to strengthen and progress their integrated commissioning and joint working further for the benefit of local people.

This solution to sustainability is also supported by organisations outside of the NHS and Local Government. For example, The Health Foundation submission to the Public Accounts Committee inquiry on sustainability and transformation in the NHS (February 2018) focussed very much upon thinking systemically and system integration. The submission identified three key ways that national bodies can support cross-organisational change:

1. Future focus is needed on what the national performance and governance frameworks should look like—they must build in the time and headspace needed to carry out redesign, allowing for experimentation and failure. This is important not just for the most advanced systems (as is currently being tested with integrated care systems) but also for those at a more formative stage of developing new models.

2. National messaging should focus on the core aims of system change and not simply on restructuring. It should encourage sites to answer the question: 'how can care be improved for patients in this area?' as opposed to 'how can this area become a new care model?'

3. Investing in robust local and national evaluation will enable sites to understand if changes are improving care. This will make sure what works and why is shared and that others can learn from their mistakes. [8, p. 5]

The case for sustainability and acute, hospital-based healthcare has been squarely located within a paradigm that uses words or phrases such as reconfiguration, integrated commissioning, integrated systems, joint working, prevention, partnerships and transformation. If sustainability is about being part of a system, then leaders from across the sectors will be reflecting upon their contributions to a system that collaborates in providing sustainable health and care?

Making Sense of Sustainability in NHS Acute Hospital Care

The term sustainability can mean different things to different people. When thinking about sustainability, it is helpful to reflect upon what we mean by the word, what is it that people are trying to achieve and in what context? For many years, NHS development organisations have provided practical guidance and support to the NHS in pursuit of the goal of sustainability.

The Sustainable Development Unit (SDU) was established and funded by NHS England and Public Health England to work across the NHS, public health and social care system. When the SDU talks about sustainability, it means helping the public sector to reduce emissions, save money and improve the health of people and communities. At an environmental level this includes addressing issues such as energy, travel, waste, procurement, water, infrastructure adaptation and the built environment. At a wider level it includes adaptation of health service delivery, health promotion, tackling the wider determinants of health, corporate social responsibility, individual responsibility and developing new sustainable models of care. (https://www.sduhealth.org.uk).

In 2013 the NHS established a Sustainability Campaign, consisting of an annual Sustainability Day. NHS and Health professionals are encouraged to "showcase how they are driving sustainability whilst celebrating their achievements and engaging with staff, patients and visitors." (https://www.nhssustainabilityday.co.uk/about-sustainability-day/). In the context of the Sustainability Campaign, sustainability means taking action in the three key areas of saving money, reducing impact on the environment and delivering higher standards of patient care.

The NHS Innovation and Improvement Agency [9] defined sustainability as follows:

Sustainability: new ways of working and improved outcomes become the norm. Not only have the process and outcome changed, but also the thinking and attitudes behind them are fundamentally altered and the systems surrounding them are transformed in support. [9, p. 9]

The NHS Institute for Innovation reported that many healthcare improvement initiatives did not continue, stating that there is evidence that one in every three improvement initiatives fails to achieve the objectives they set out to. The implications of this failure rate are compromised patient experience, a waste of resources, finances, staff time and a risk to their future engagement in opportunities to transform services [9, p. 25]. Two major challenges were identified:

1. The improvement evaporation effect or initiative decay. This is what happens when an improvement has been implemented but is not

embedded into the organisations 'business as usual' and things reverts to how they were before change was made.

2. Isolated improvements or improvement islands. This is what happens when an improvement is sustained within a team or service area, but doesn't spread more widely through the organisation or across other organisations [9, p. 8]

Figure 12.1, produced by NHS I&I [9], illustrates key enablers that should exist within organisations aiming to sustain improvement.

In order to provide organisations with a practical tool, the NHS I&I [10] developed a Sustainability Model and Guide. The guide states that the most successful organisations are those that can implement and sustain effective improvement initiatives which lead to increased quality and patient experience at lower cost. The Sustainability Model aims to identify strengths and weaknesses in implementation plans and predict the likelihood of a sustainable improvement initiative. The model, illustrated by the NHS I&I in Fig. 12.2, identifies the main factors affecting sustainability of an improvement initiative and groups them under the three themes of staff, process and organisation. Each theme has several associated factors against which organisations or teams can self-assess the likelihood of implementing an improvement and of sustaining any change.

The Model was not designed to assess whether a department, whole organisation or health community is likely to sustain an innovation or transformational change. It was recommended that its use should be linked to a specific improvement project or initiative. The model supports the implementation of change and in so doing recognises that, at project or system level, any improvement is dependent upon change as an essential component for sustainability. As new evidence emerges, and clinical practices change with new technologies or medicines, then a continuation of a new way of working is less important than an organisations ability to constantly adapt or to transform when today's change becomes yesterday's way of doing things.

It is clear that sustainability has many dimensions that range from implementing a small-scale project to the transformation of the way an organisation delivers its services through to how a system might continue to be financially viable, reduce its environmental impact and improve the quality of care for an entire population. At the level of, for example, an acute hospital trust, we suggest that sustainability requires the organisation to focus upon their capacity and capability to continually change. However, organisations work within a complex and multi-faceted system of health and care that requires the sum of all the parts of the system to collaborate in order to collectively adapt to economic, political, social and

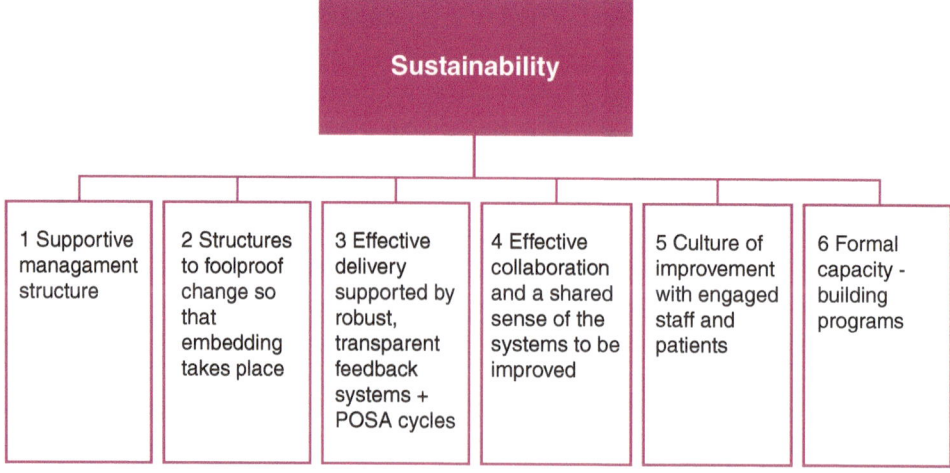

Fig. 12.1 Key enablers for sustainable improvement [9, p. 18]

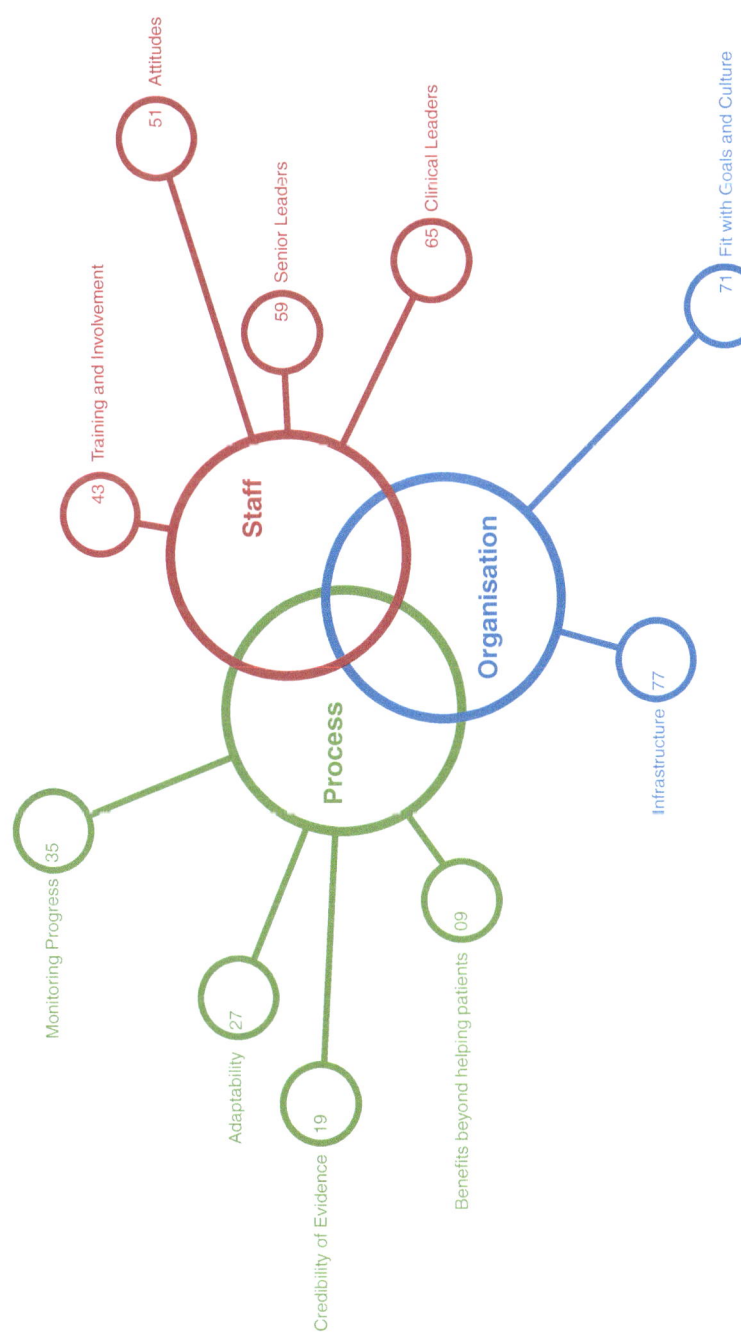

Fig. 12.2 The NHS Innovation and Improvement model for sustainability [10]

environmental changes. Sustainability requires leaders to think 'whole system' and how they can overcome challenges that mitigate against working in this way.

What Can We Learn from Other Health Systems?

Dougall et al. [11] have described and reviewed four organisations who have been recognised for their place-based transformation work: The Bromley by Bow Centre in East London; Birmingham and Solihull Mental Health Trust, Northumbria Health care NHS Foundation Trust and Buurtzorg (from the Netherlands). The review draws out a number of key challenges the systems faced:

1. *Overcoming inertia—creating a receptive context*
   Staff were very engaged and motivated by improving care, but many people did not feel able to act as change leaders
2. *The concept of power*
   'Power' was important in the transformational change stories, sometimes as a barrier that could often be disempowering. But, where power was shared it became empowering
3. *'Old power' and 'new power'*
   Power dynamics were important in the stories. For example, 'old power' held by the few and closely guarded versus 'new power', enabling people at grassroots level to exercise agency. There were some examples of the shift from old to new power.
4. *Maintain dual focus*
   Working effectively within current constraints, whilst championing fundamentally different structures and approaches to support transformation was challenging but that a dual focus is needed
5. *Difficult choices*
   There were tensions between radical innovation and the need to protect people from harm, between the pace of change and the time it takes to fully engage people, the balance between providing acute are compared to having a longer term preventative focus.

Baker [12] reviewed a small group of high performing healthcare systems: Jonkoping County Council, Intermountain Healthcare, Henry Ford Health System and VA New England Healthcare System. Baker identified ten key themes underlying the sustainability of the care systems:

1. *Consistent leadership that embraces common goals and aligns activities throughout the organisation*
   The systems had strong senior leadership, but leadership in the systems was also distributed and collective
2. *Quality and system improvement as a core strategy*
   Transformation was a slow process, so a clear and sustained strategy over time was important
3. *Organisational capacities and skills to support performance improvement*
   Consistent effort was made to enhance skills and capabilities among staff and to change the vision that drives provision of services
4. *Robust primary care teams at the centre of the delivery system*
   Integrated, effective primary care was a vital part of creating a better performing health care system overall
5. *Engaging patients in their care and in design of care*
   Whole person care, comprehensive communication and coordination, patient support and empowerment
6. *Promoting professional cultures that support teamwork, continuous improvement and patient engagement*
   A real commitment to building a professional culture that encourages and regards improvement, patient engagement and teamwork.
7. *More effective integration of care that promotes seamless care transitions*
   Recognising the interdependence between system levels means that quality improvement must also improve transitions of care between the parts of the system

8. *Information   as   a   platform   guiding improvement*

Focus on identifying and measurement to support improvement, with local teams collecting their own measures of clinical performance to track their progress toward clinical goals

9. *Effective learning strategies and methods to test improvements and scale up*

Close linkages with other organisations, and have proactively identified new methods and tools and adapted them to local environments.

10. *Providing an enabling environment buffering short-term factors that undermine success*

All the systems have faced major challenges, but achieved by adopting a long-term strategy for improving care, working to develop talent and create a focus on providing patient centred care.

Collaboration and Working in Partnership

As well as considering the transformation project itself, leaders will understand how to work in partnership within an individual organisation and also across a system. The health and care system is a complex environment, with many competing demands and pressures. This environment can thwart the most promising transformation projects and working in partnership is a particular skill, even when the transformation remains within a single organisation.

Collaboration Within the Organisation

Whilst an organisation is a single entity, it is our observation that how well the organisation cooperates internally is a significant factor in (a) how well an organisation can initiate improvement or transformation projects and (b) how well they will sustain them. This is because many projects are not contained within one team or department. Therefore, if there isn't an organisational culture of working together to solve a common problem, sustainability of transformation across the organisational will be a struggle.

Much has been written about organisational culture in the NHS, which we won't discuss here, except to say that organisational culture is a significant factor in the sustainability of transformation. If directorates or departments are encouraged and incentivised to compete against each other, even in seemingly innocuous ways, then working together on a change or transformation project will be so much harder. For example, the sustainability of tackling the pressures faced by Accident and Emergency Departments will stand a greater chance of success if the Hospital is able to transfer people onto an appropriate ward by creating space through reducing the length of stays in the Hospital. This could then require, for example, initiatives that facilitate the timely resolution of any diagnostic tests and the prompt prescribing of medicines to enable earlier discharge.

There is a real challenge for leaders of organisations to implement what they consider 'rigorous' performance management, whilst not creating negative side effects. There is nothing like competition between teams to create an insidious culture where teams cannot look beyond their own boundary to support transformation projects.

Collaboration Outside the Organisation

Fragmentation and competition within a health system is not suited to solving the complex challenges that all health systems are facing. This is now broadly recognised, and a significant shift in language can been seen across policy documents and health committee reviews. It is recognised that health incorporates mental, physical and social wellbeing and many factors contribute to good health such as quality housing, education, employment, community networks and others [13]. Indeed, the direction of travel in the NHS is very much on partnerships and integrated care systems.

This approach provides a significant psychological challenge to sovereign organisations that have survived thus far by competing with their peers. It requires leaders to work together, spanning boundaries between organisations whilst prioritising patient care, rather than the success of their organisation or component of the system [14]. The complexity of transformation projects in these circumstances is infinitely greater, especially if the individual organisations have a competitive culture and struggle to cooperate internally. However, more integrated and system wide approaches can be achieved and there are excellent initiatives across the UK where commissioners, primary care, acute sector providers, social care and the independent sector have collaborated to ensure the timely discharge of people from hospital back into their own homes or into intermediate care services.

Genuine partnership approaches that engage the whole of the system are essential when facing the challenges of most health and care systems [15]. Both leaders and organisations have been rewarded for working competitively for decades and are now required to work differently. They are required to work collectively and build a cooperative, integrative leadership culture—in effect, collective leadership at the system level [16]. In addition, there is the challenge of statutory legislation which requires them to compete as service providers, which in part is a genuine barrier, but can also be used as a convenient 'excuse' to maintain the status quo.

Working collaboratively across systems is required to address 'wicked' problems, but collaboration is not easy when the health and care system remains fragmented and regulators can often operate inconsistently. In working across systems, we have observed the power of individual leaders who possess excellent skills in building positive relationships and adopt pragmatic, yet effective approaches when negotiating system wide barriers such as competition. Senge et al. [17] conclude that transforming systems is ultimately about transforming relationships among people who shape those systems.

A themed review by the NIHR Dissemination Centre [18], entitled *Advancing Care: Research with care homes*, concluded that the research evidence clearly supports partnership working between care homes, the NHS and wider stakeholders at individual, organisational and system levels. Determined efforts to build and maintain positive working relationships were identified as a key enabler for the success and sustainability of health and wellbeing improvement initiatives in care homes for older people. It is our experience that failure to value and transform relationships often leads to change efforts failing or not being sustained.

How to Work Across a System

The evidence from other integrated care systems confirms the importance of the time needed to build relationships to establish quality efforts towards local transformation [11, 14, 17, 19]. Hulks et al. [20] have drawn upon the work of Michael West and others, and identified five factors that facilitate working across systems:

1. *Develop a shared purpose and vision*
   This requires a shift from reactive problem-solving to building positive visions for the future. This includes confronting difficult choices about the present reality as part of working towards an inspiring vision
2. *Have frequent personal contact*
   Collaboration is a team activity, a contact sport that cannot be conducted at distance. It requires leadership to establish the rapport and understanding as a basis for a collaborative relationship
3. *Surface and resolve conflicts*
   Collaboration is not easy nor straightforward. Agreements will go hand in hand with disagreements. If they are allowed to fester and undermine relationships and trust, disagreements can be fatal to collaboration.
4. *Behave altruistically towards each other*
   Leaders who are now seeking to collaborate with each other, will have often found themselves competing in the past. This means moving from a win-lose style of negotiation to win-win.
5. *Commit to working together for the longer term*
   This matters because of the investment of time and energy needed to build effective relationships.

The nature of health care provision in the NHS has changed significantly over the last few years with a move towards system thinking. This means understanding how working in partnership will ensure that a transformation is sustained. As the NHS is trying to operate more as a system, rather than a collection of individual organisations, recognising the impact of the environment and context must be considered in relation to any transformation.

Environment and Context

Understanding Context

Ensuring that transformation is sustainable starts at the early planning stage. At the outset of any transformation, it is time well spent to understand the type of problem or challenges that any change is seeking to address. Different types of challenges need different approaches, both in terms of leadership style and the solution design. This is commonly overlooked, with one style of approach being used across different challenges for which it is not appropriate.

By working in partnership, it offers leaders an opportunity to rethink and to create completely different, more effective ways of addressing challenges [11]. Working across an organisation or system is however more complex and provides a very different operating context for leaders. When working in a complex environment with little certainty, linear cause and effect models are not appropriate, and a flexible approach is required [21].

Working in a complex environment provides a series of often paradoxical challenges for leaders. To work successfully in a system, leaders must have a good understanding of context and the ability to embrace complexity and paradox. There are frameworks that support leaders operating in complex environments to address real world challenges (e.g. [22]). The Cynefin framework offers a way to understand different contexts [22]. Snowdon has tested and applied the framework in different leadership contexts, sectors and environments to identify the leadership styles that were most successful in the different contexts.

The Cynefin Framework [23] summarises the different contexts and leadership approaches. It provides a clear way of categorising the context of the challenge or problem that a transformation is intended to address. In our experience, very little effort is put into really understanding and defining the problem that is trying to be solved. The same is true of defining success measures. We have often found very little relationship between the problem that is trying to be solved and what 'good' looks like. Without a clear, rational line of thought from start to end, often well-meant transformation and improvement initiatives end up being confusing in their ambition and tend not to meet the expectations of all stakeholders. This can then lead to those involved in such programs to be disillusioned and less likely to put psychological effort and physical commitment into transformation projects in the future.

Cynefin, pronounced ku-nev-in, is a Welsh word that signifies 'place' or 'habitat', but also the multiple factors in our environment [22]. Context is a significant factor which should shape the response to the problem, a one size fits all response is not an effective approach. The Cynefin framework identifies five cause and effect domains: complex; complicated; chaotic; simple; disorder. A few words on each context are below.

Simple Context The simple context is when there are 'known—knowns' to address the problem. For example, we know that anti-coagulating patients with atrial fibrillation will reduce their risk of stroke. Simple does not mean easy, but there is a cause and effect relationship, it is likened to following a recipe.

Complicated Context In this context there may be several potential solutions, so some testing and adjusting is required. It is likened to sending a rocket into space, much is known but there is still some testing and input from experts required.

Complex Context In this context little is known, there are many 'unknown-unkowns' which means to address problems in this context, a testing approach is required. It is likened to raising a child, as what works in one situation may not work in another and generalising is often not possible.

Chaotic Context In this context there is no relationship between cause and effect, the priority is to establish order and stability. Crisis and emergency scenarios often fall into this domain e.g. the attack on the Twin Towers in New York.

Disorder When it isn't clear which of the other four domains is dominant, you are in a 'disorder' situation.

It is possible for a problem to move through different domains, starting as 'complicated' and becoming 'simple'. As highlighted earlier, an example of a complex challenge is improving the performance and outcomes of NHS urgent and emergency care departments. For many years the NHS urgent and emergency care services have been under pressure with continued growth in levels of emergency admissions and from delayed transfers of care when patients require admission to a hospital ward or are ready to leave hospital. NHS England led the development of a national programme of activities designed to improve the urgent and emergency care (UEC) system so patients "get the right care in the right place, whenever they need it".

A number of different interventions were identified that could have an impact on the quality and effectiveness of care. It is the task of local leaders to collaborate and take a 'system leadership' role with partners and to co-ordinate a program of interventions that, collectively, aimed to reduce the pressures upon the UEC system. Examples from an English Sustainable Transformation Partnership (STP) included:

- Using quality improvement methods when supporting A & E departments to improve patient flow within a hospital.
- Integrating and analysing data from an Ambulance Service, 111 and an NHS out of hours service provider to re-design care

pathways that improve patient flow through out of hours services.
- Implementing a community pharmacy project designed to reduce prescribing demand on out of hours GP services
- Implementing an out of hours direct booking initiative designed to enable NHS 111 services to book appointments directly into GP practices.
- Implementing a Clinical Advisory Service (CAS) to provide care navigation and clinical advice to 111, 999 & front line healthcare professionals
- Ensuring the coordinated development and provision of urgent treatment centres

It is often the case in health and social care that there are multiple initiatives happening at the same time and these can be locally, regionally or nationally led. It can be difficult to see how they fit together and how their impact might be evaluated, not as individual projects but upon, for example, the operations of an urgent and emergency care system of multiple interventions and involving multiple care providers and commissioners.

Taking one of the initiatives cited as an example, implementing an out of hours booking initiative to enable NHS 111 services to book appointments directly into GP practices. If patients have been triaged by NHS 111 and categorised as not immediately urgent, they would not be offered an appointment with an out of hours doctor. However, it was found to be the case that many patients would attend A&E as a default way to receive an appointment more quickly. The initiative was designed to reduce attendance at A & E by NHS 111 directly booking an appointment with the patient's GP for the next day, thus reducing uncertainty for patients when they will be seen by a doctor.

The multiplicity of stakeholders, IT systems and independent processes are complicated. The GP practices, 111 and NHS GP out of hours services are all managed separately, have different IT systems and different approaches to managing their appointments. A cause and effect relationship can be hypothesised, and the outcome is potentially knowable. However, it is not entirely predictable as there are multiple variables that could impact upon the outcome. For example, would people who contact services be prepared to wait until the next day for a GP appointment?

Expert knowledge is required to ensure that different IT systems can support the changes. Workforce training and support is required to ensure that that call handlers are aware of how they can directly book into GP practices. GPs will need to be satisfied that the changes are safe, that the 111 triage process is robust and does not allow people to inappropriately receive a GP appointment. When implementing this project, there are 'known unknowns' and therefore, according to the Cynefin framework, this could be categorised as a complicated project. The project cannot be a 'complex' project as there is a proposed solution to a problem. Whilst it may not necessarily be the correct solution, there is a hypothesis and a way to progress the project. Only when starting to deliver the project will it become clear whether the assumptions were correct. Of course, the model is open to interpretation, but it does provide a helpful starting point. If things aren't progressing as you would have liked, you can use the model to review and then try a different approach.

At an individual level, the Direct Booking project might be complicated. However, at the same time, NHS England has been supporting the transformation of Urgent and Emergency Care (UEC) services through the development of what has been called a Consolidated Channel Shift Model. This model aims to connect UEC services together, so the overall system becomes more than just the sum of its parts. This has entailed identifying a number of separate interventions, delivered by different organisations across a local UEC health economy. The interventions were designed to shift activity away from hospital based Accident and Emergency centres to the most appropriate setting of care. The model is underpinned by a belief that there is no single intervention or activity that will ease the pressure on UEC services and it is the combined effect of several interventions, across different parts of the system, that makes the difference. This approach to the combined effect of interventions must be considered as a system change.

If the Direct Booking project is 'nested' within a wider transformation programme that covers multiple health economies across an STP footprint, then the leadership challenge moves from complicated to complex. The cause and effect relationships are unlikely to be repeatable as each local health economy and each STP footprint has a different configuration of services with varying levels of capacity and access thresholds. The collective impact of the transformation is likely to reveal emergent patterns that are unique to the locality and to the STP footprint and, as a consequence, interventions will need to be further adjusted and tested to achieve the desired results. Unexpected consequences are more likely to emerge as organisations and people accessing services all respond differently to the multiple service changes that have been introduced.

Using this framework to understand the context of the transformation or improvement challenge increases the likelihood of the transformation being sustained. This is because an understanding of the context of the challenge will assist in understanding the most appropriate approach to take and, furthermore, it helps to define the leadership behaviours required in each context. It is important to note that problems move domains, so it is the job of leaders to create an adaptive approach and supporting systems to enable differential responses throughout the life of the project.

Context and Leadership Behaviours

As well as defining the context to help us understand the transformation or challenges, Snowdon and Boone [22] identify different leadership responses to apply to the different contexts.

This is helpful to leaders as it clearly defines how to respond to each context. When we first came across this framework, we could see why the broad brush, eye watering statistics of change efforts fail. Inevitably, any organisation or system will have problems in all domains at different times. This is why one approach to transformation does not fit all situations and why an adaptive approach to transformation and the leadership styles applied is critical to ensure the problem is addressed and is more likely to be sustained in the future.

It is easy to see why many of the transformation or improvement projects don't sustain. There is an understandable tendency for senior managers, civil servants and policy makers to create change projects that use 'fact based management'. We feel more comfortable when we think we understand things (in a simple context), using a cause and effect approach. We tend to like a sense of control for our actions. We also tend to work in an operational culture where failure is perceived to be exactly that, a failure rather an opportunity to learn. Working in the complex context, it is much less clear to determine what should be done, how it should be done and how to predict the outcome or impact. A series of trial and error actions must be undertaken to try and determine the preferred course of action that will result in the desired impact.

Our experience is that engaging staff in the definition of the problem, as well as the creation and implementation of the solution is the most effective approach to achieving sustainable change. Again, this is an area for improvement across the NHS and public sector. Having evidence to define the problem and to shape the development of a solution is important, but it is often not enough when aiming to sustain any change. We all know that change can be difficult for people and, as you might expect, supporting and leading change is more complex... or is it complicated?

The Type of Change and How to Deliver It

As well as understanding the context of the problem that you are trying to solve, it is important to understand the barriers to behaviour change. The change strategy must address barriers to behaviour change, otherwise it is unlikely that the change will be achieved or sustained [24]. There are many behaviour change theories which we are not discussing in this chapter, but the most useful ones in relation to achieving change are those that have been developed from a strong evidence base and have been applied in many contexts. The Behaviour Change Wheel (BCW) [25] enables leaders to design interventions and achieve behaviour change in complex situations. The BCW was developed from 19 frameworks of behaviours identified in a systematic literature review. It consists of three layers as indicated in Fig. 12.3 below.

The behaviour change wheel helps you to understand which behaviours may need to be targeted to achieve the transformation objective. It uses the COM-B model of behaviour change. The model explains there are three different behavioural elements to address and to achieve change, these are: Capability, Opportunity & Motivation, as indicated in Fig. 12.4 below.

In order to achieve change, transformation projects should understand which behaviours to target and how they should be changed. This is important to ensure that any behaviour change is sustained, and that individuals don't revert back to their previous behaviour(s).

Surrounding the three core elements in the hub, is a layer of nine interventions functions to select, depending on the initial COM-B analysis undertaken. The outer layer then identified seven policy categories that can support the delivery of these new behaviours as part of the transformation program. As the context can change depending on the stage of the project, it is important to note that the behaviour change interventions may also have to change, depending on the path of the project and any unexpected influences.

When designing any transformation project, it is important to follow a systematic approach that allows an intervention to achieve behaviour change to be developed. Working in this way will mean a higher likelihood of the new behaviour happening and being sustained. This is the value of using a framework like this, as it helps identify the intervention to use to achieve the greatest chance of achieving behaviour change.

The COM-B model of behaviour change helps you further understand the nature of

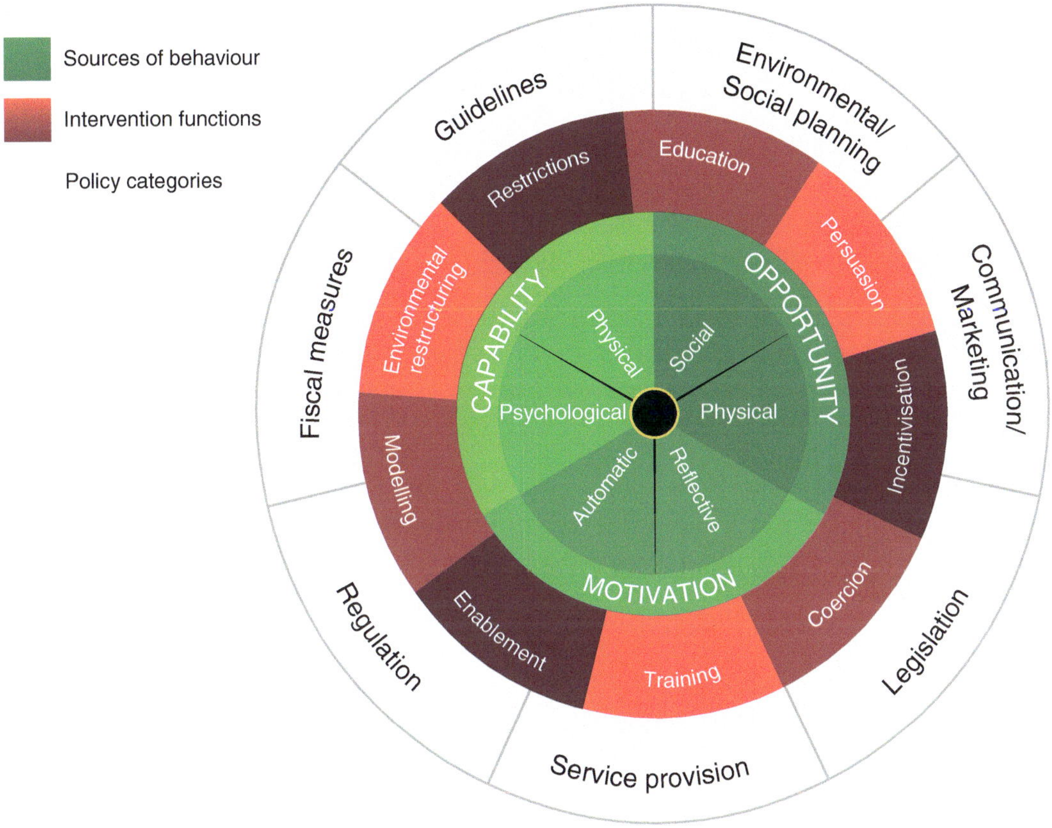

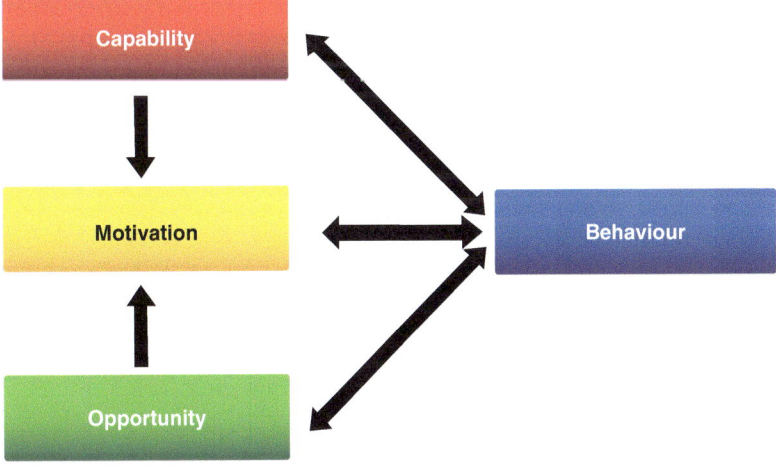

Fig. 12.3 The behaviour change wheel [25]

Fig. 12.4 The COM-B system—a framework for understanding behaviour [25]

the actions to be taken to achieve behaviour change. The model suggests that for any behaviour to occur an individual must have the physical and psychological capability to perform the behaviour, the social and physical opportunity and be motivated to perform the target behaviour more than any other behaviour. Having the physical ability and stamina to ride a bicycle is an example of the capability to perform. Understanding the factors that form part of behaviours is important because it helps define which behaviours, or factors influencing behaviour lie within the person (e.g. the capability to ride a bicycle) and which lie outside the individual (e.g. availability of cycle paths).

The outer ring of the behaviour change wheel identifies the range of interventions that could be used as potential levers of change. Table 12.1 links between the components of the COM-B model of behaviour and the intervention functions in the Behaviour Change Wheel that are required to support change [25].

Different interventions can be chosen depending on the impact required. As projects can change in their nature, from complex to complicated for example, so too can the interventions required to sustain the desired change in behaviour.

It is important to acknowledge the dynamic relationship that exists between the context of the change that is taking place and the barriers and opportunities presented by cross-boundary working. Focussing on relationships and communication is important, particularly when working in a complex system. Understanding the barriers to behaviour change is essential, as is recognising that whilst rules, protocols, directives or performance targets have their place in achieving a change in behaviour, they are not the critical tools that we often believe them to be. This is important for those leading change programs of this nature; the importance of modelling system leadership behaviours cannot be underestimated.

Conclusion and Key Messages

Defining sustainability is multi-faceted and can mean different things to different people. People will behave differently depending upon their roles as, for example, a finance director, a patient, a clinician or an environmentalist. This chapter has focussed on four key areas for NHS leaders seeking to undertake sustainable

transformation: understanding context, system thinking, collaboration and facilitating behaviour change. We have described some tools that can help navigate what is often very confusing territory in an informed and structured way. The key points that we would like to highlight are:

1. Leadership can and should come from anybody, not only those in formal positions of authority.
   - To ensure transformation is sustained, there must be a good number of advocates capable of adapting to change, maintaining momentum, ensuring delivery and evaluating impact.
2. Creating structures and mechanisms that facilitate more collaborative and integrated working.
   - Build a collaborative infrastructure that encourage collaboration, example genuinely shared vision, values and goals and outcomes are really important to help individuals understand that sustainability is not just about the success of leaders' individual areas of responsibility
3. Don't underestimate the influence of context and environment upon the sustainable transformation of services
4. Work across systems for transformation to be sustainable
   - No single organisation or department 'is an island'
5. Understand the behavioural barriers and enablers to sustainability and focus effort and energy on these right from the beginning.
6. Working across complex systems requires the testing of multiple approaches
   - Systematically implement quality improvement methods, learn from 'failed' approaches and allow success to emerge.
7. The ability to create and maintain constructive, effective relationships underpins all the above points.
   - Without positive relationships, achieving everything else is so much harder.

Table 12.1 Linking the COM-B model to the Behaviour Change Wheel

COM B component	Intervention Function								
	education	Persuasion	Incentivisation	Coercion	Training	Restriction	Environmental restructuring	Modelling	Enablement
Physical capability	X				X				X
Psychological capability					X				X
Physical opportunity					X	X	X		X
Social opportunity						X	X	X	X
Automatic motivation		X	X	X	X		X	X	X
Reflective motivation	X	X	X	X					

References

1. NHS England. NHS five year forward view. 2014. https://www.england.nhs.uk/five-year-forward-view/. Accessed 29 Mar 2018.
2. CQC. The state of care in NHS acute hospitals: 2014 to 2016 findings from the end of CQC's programme of NHS acute comprehensive inspections. 2017. Available at https://www.cqc.org.uk/sites/default/files/20170302b_stateofhospitals_web.pdf. Accessed 20 July 2018.
3. NHS England. Next steps on the NHS five year forward view. 2017. Available at https://tinyurl.com/mfl4td7. Accessed 29 June 2018.
4. Ham C, Alderwick H, Dunn P, McKenna H. Delivering sustainability and transformation plans from ambitious proposals to credible plans. London: The Kings Fund; 2017. https://www.kingsfund.org.uk/sites/default/files/field/field_publication_file/STPs_proposals_to_plans_Kings_Fund_Feb_2017_0.pdf.
5. NHS Improvement. Plan, do study act cycles and the model for improvement. 2018. https://improvement.nhs.uk/resources/pdsa-cycles/. Accessed 28 June 2018.
6. National Audit Office. Report by the Controller and Auditor General Ministry of Housing, Communities & Local Government Financial sustainability of local authorities. 2018. Available at https://www.nao.org.uk/wp-content/uploads/2018/03/Financial-sustainabilty-of-local-authorites-2018.pdf. Accessed 23 Aug 2018.
7. Local Government Association. Integrated commissioning for better outcomes: a commissioning framework. 2018. Available at www.local.gov.uk/sites/default/files/documents/25.70_Integrated%20Commissioning%20for%20Better%20Outcomes_final.pdf. Accessed 25 June 2018.
8. The Health Foundation. Submission: public accounts committee inquiry on sustainability and transformation in the NHS. London: The Health Foundation; 2018. Available at https://www.health.org.uk/sites/health/files/Health%20Foundation%20submission%20-%20PAC%20sustainability%20and%20transformation%20in%20the%20NHS.pdf. Accessed 28 June 2018.
9. NHS Institute for Innovation and Improvement. Improvement leaders' guide sustainability and its relationship with spread and adoption. 2007. Available at https://www.england.nhs.uk/improvement-hub/publication/improvement-leaders-guide-sustainability-and-its-relationship-with-spread-and-adoption-general-improvement-skills/. Accessed 28 June 2018.
10. NHS Institute for Innovation and Improvement. Sustainability model and guide. 2010. Available at https://www.england.nhs.uk/improvement-hub/wp-content/uploads/sites/44/2017/11/NHS-Sustainability-Model-2010.pdf.
11. Dougall D, Lewis M, Ross S. Transformational change in health and care. Reports from the field. London: The King's Fund; 2018. Available at https://www.kingsfund.org.uk/publications/transformational-change-health-care Accessed 10 May 2018.
12. Baker GR. The roles of leaders in high-performing health care systems. London: The King's Fund; 2011. Available at https://www.kingsfund.org.uk/publications/articles/roles-leaders-high-performing-health-care-systems Accessed 4 Mar 2018.
13. Buck D. Housing: a home for STPs looking to influence the wider determinants of health. Blog. The King's Fund website. 2018. Available at www.kingsfund.org.uk/blog/2018/03/housing-stps-wider-determinants-health Accessed on 19 April 2018.
14. West M, Armit K, Loewenthal L, Eckert R, West T, Lee A. Leadership and leadership development in health care: the evidence base. London: The King's Fund & Centre for Creative Leadership; 2015. Available at https://www.kingsfund.org.uk/sites/default/files/field/field_publication_file/leadership-leadership-development-health-care-feb-2015.pdf. Accessed 15 Mar 2018.
15. Ham C. Whole system transformation requires whole-system engagement. Blog. The King's Fund Website. 2017. Available at https://www.kingsfund.org.uk/blog/2017/10/whole-system-transformation-needs-whole-system-engagement. Accessed 1 Apr 2018.
16. Savigny D, Adam T, editors. Systems thinking for health systems strengthening. Geneva: Alliance for Health Policy and Systems Research. World Health Organisation; 2009.
17. Senge P, Hamilton H, Kania J. The dawn of system leadership. Stanf Soc Innov Rev. 2015;13(1):27–33. Available at https://ssir.org/articles/entry/the_dawn_of_system_leadership Accessed 10 Mar 2018.
18. NIHR Dissemination Centre. Advancing care: research with care homes Themed Review. 2017. https://www.dc.nihr.ac.uk/themed-reviews/advancing-care-themed-review.pdf
19. Timmins N. The practice of system leadership, being comfortable with chao. London: The King's Fund; 2015. Available at https://www.kingsfund.org.uk/publications/practice-system-leadership. Accessed on 4 Apr 2018.
20. Hulks S, Walsh N, Powell M, Ham C, Alderwick H. Leading across the health and care system, lessons from experience. London: The King's Fund; 2017. Available at https://www.kingsfund.org.uk/publications/leading-across-health-and-care-system.
21. Plsek P, Greenhalgh T. The challenge of complexity in health care. Br Med J. 2001;232:625–8.
22. Snowden DJ, Boone ME. A leader's framework for decision making. Harv Bus Rev. 2007;85(11):69–76.
23. Snowden D. Cynefin framework. 2019. Available at https://cognitive-edge.com/sensemaker/. Accessed 12 Jan 2019.
24. Mitchie S, West R, Campbell R, Brown J, Gainforth HL. ABC of behaviour change theories. London: Silverback Publishing; 2014.
25. Mitchie S, van Stralen MM, West R. The behaviour change wheel: a new method for characterising and designing behaviour change interventions. Implement Sci. 2011;6(1):1.

Andrew Cash

The 1948 National Health Service (NHS): 'In Place of Fear'

Seventy years ago almost to the day that I write this, if you were living in England, a leaflet would have come through your letterbox promising you the new National Health Service. And in beautifully clear prose it states:

> The new National Health Service begins on 5 July 1948. What it is, how do you get it?

The leaflet says 'it will provide you with all medical, dental and nursing care, everyone rich or poor, man, woman or child can use it or any part of it. There are no charges except for a few special items, there are no insurance qualifications. But it is not a charity. You are all paying for it. Mainly as tax payers. And it will relieve your money worries in times of illness' [1].

The National Health Service (NHS) was the first universal healthcare system developed after the Second World War and was founded 'in place of fear'. After the trauma of the war years, people demanded a new set of arrangements across a number of public services and the NHS was designed to provide essentially free care, at the point of need, irrespective of age, health, race, religion, social status or the ability to pay—from 'cradle to the grave'.

A. Cash (✉)
Sheffield Teaching Hospitals NHS Foundation Trust, Sheffield, UK

Recommitting to the NHS: Why Do We Do It?

To most people in England the creation of the NHS is considered one of the proudest achievements of modern society representing fairness and equity, held dear by all. Yet an underlying paranoia about the NHS remains. About once a decade in the subsequent years since its creation in 1948 we have as a country decided whether to recommit to that conception of a national health service. Indeed it is pretty easy to forget that the health service was born at a time of great economic austerity, in the post-war period when there was no great reason for thinking, other than a great spirit of optimism, that the economic wherewith-all would be there to support this huge endeavour.

Nye Bevan who, of course, founded the NHS in 1948 said 'this is the biggest single experiment in social service that the world has ever seen' [2].

He also reminded everybody at the tenth anniversary of the NHS in 1958 that one of the great difficulties in 1948 was that mass radiography was just beginning to detect early tuberculosis (TB) so there was a huge expansion required for TB beds and treatment. Thirty two thousand beds in the NHS were occupied by people with TB on the day it was founded. And one of the main reasons why we had a particular problem with the beds was that we could not recruit enough nurses. Bevan said at the time 'they were so inadequately paid and the conditions were so bad that they could not recruit enough nurses in sufficient numbers, indeed' he said 'I myself had to take the unusual step of intervening in negotiations to secure an increase in the wages for nurses' [3].

Of course the inception of the NHS was bitterly opposed by many people but despite that context, despite the capacity shortages, the NHS came into being and is now the most treasured institution in our country. So it is very heartening to hear the Prime Minister, Theresa May, just a few weeks before the 70th birthday of the NHS, once again, recommit her government to a multi year funding settlement for the NHS for the next 10 years.

So why do we keep recommitting to the NHS? Well, costing an average of £6.16 p per person per day, it is a tremendous economical bargain for the people of this country and relieves the anxiety of not being able to afford healthcare when you need it. BUT of course it is more than that—the NHS is a people business—a mixture of care and compassion on the one hand and incredible science and technology on the other. OK, it can seem large, bureaucratic and complex at times but at its most simplest, it is about two people together, one needing help and the other offering it.

Overcoming the Challenges: Lessons from History

The issue we now face is will the NHS, designed 70 years ago, still be fit to tackle the challenges we face ahead? Moreover what do we need to do to make sure the NHS is fit for purpose for the next 5, 10, 15 and 20 years?

History tells us that the world of healthcare is constantly evolving around that basic construct of care and compassion and the person receiving treatment and the person giving it. Science and technology is advancing. People are finding better ways of doing things. Whether it is in the field of information technology, the electronic patient record or artificial intelligence or in the way we manage buildings and services. Or in new and innovative approaches to workforce development

or different national policy changes in leadership from competition to collaboration. One thing is clear, this country has a rich track record of success.

On science and technology alone, picture a country that had made a global impact on medical and health care science. A country that had invented a vaccination for smallpox, that discovered the first antibiotics, performed the first stem cell transplant and invented in-vitro fertilisation.

Or on medical devices, a country that had invented the thermometer, the artificial hip, the MRI and the CT scanner.

Or a country that punched well above its weight in terms of medical research with 1% of the worlds population but 16% of the worlds highest cited research papers. Putting all these sorts of achievements together gives you the ability to create a wonderful health and care system—and all these elements exist here, in this country—and in the NHS.

So in this simple example of science and innovation, we are able to see one of the endearing strengths of the NHS in England. That is the relationship between academic research and clinical practice. According to the Times Higher Education World University Rankings, England has three of the top five worldwide universities for clinical, pre-clinical and health subjects and has four universities in the top ten across all subjects [4]. The UK is placed second for hosting the largest number of clinical trials after the US and, in absolute terms, fourth in the world for health research behind the US, Japan and Germany [5].

The New Challenges

Living Longer

When the NHS was set up in 1948 the average life expectancy of a male was just over 65 years and slightly more for females. Half the male population was dead by retirement age. Now it is just over 82 years for males and slightly more for females. Our population is very different. We have an increasingly ageing population with people regularly living into their 80s and 90s. And there is a spectrum of health—some people are hugely active, others require help from time to time at home. At the other end of the spectrum are those that require considerable intervention and support.

Changing Expectations

People are far better informed about their health, their own conditions, treatment and care needs. More and more carers look after and support loved ones, and more and more people need to be supported in developing the knowledge, skills and confidence to manage their own conditions and to care for others. Increasingly people want to stay active and be prescribed exercise as a way forward.

Shortages in the Workforce

Developing a sustainable healthcare workforce is the key foundation stone required for a successful health and care system and is integral to the quality and safety of the service provided, particularly in the light of Brexit and an uncertain future. More people want flexible careers, reflecting generational expectations and recognising this in the way we attract, recruit and retain staff in the future is the number one challenge we face.

Technology and Innovation

Predicting how health and care will change in the next 5 years, let alone 20, in the face of technological change and innovation is exciting but tricky to assess. What we do know is ready access to information and genomic medicine, for example, will radically shape and change how we deliver services in the future. We will see the growth of precision medicine, robotics and portable digital diagnostic devices changing how patients, carers and staff use and access services in the future.

Integrating Health and Care

Both the health and social care sectors are completely interdependent with both sectors facing similar demographic and population challenges. Many people receiving care and treatment in the health sector are very often experiencing a 'social care 'crisis but have ended up in the health world and visa versa.

Changing Socio-Economic Environment

Recognising the social determinants of health—choice, education, your job, housing etc.—and doing something about them, have long been recognised as the 'holy grail' to improving health inequalities and improving health outcomes for everyone, not just the few. The social and political leadership required to tackle these thorny issues over a lengthier period of time than just the normal 5 year government cycle is the key. Changing the language of health from 'illness' to 'prevention 'requires as a starter a change in long term economic resource allocation.

Overcoming the Challenges: the New NHS Leadership Task

So if Nye Bevan were here today and starting the NHS anew to overcome these challenges, what would he do?

Leading Through Organising Services Around Individuals

Firstly, we need to acknowledge that whilst it is great that we are living longer, we need to understand that many more of us will develop multiple long term conditions (stroke, diabetes, heart disease etc). Here are some key facts—11.6 million people in England are aged 65 and over, an increase of 21% in a decade whilst 1.5 million are aged 85 or over, an increase of 31% over the same period. 3.8 million people live with diabetes, 2.5 million have a cancer diagnosis and one million additional people will have dementia by 2021. Leaders need to build services and care around individuals not the other way around as has been the NHS pattern of delivery in the past [6].

Integrating Health and Care Services

Secondly, we need to back the leadership of the newly formed Sustainability and Transformation Partnerships across the country and as they mature, the new Integrated Care Systems (ICS's). Each ICS covering a geographical population footprint ideally of 1.5 million people or above needs to get its constituent hospitals, care organisations, social service sectors, ambulance services, clinical commissioning groups, primary care federations, voluntary and third sector organisations to work together. This is so that they can improve health inequalities for the population, to provide equality of access to high quality services for all residents and to achieve the best value for money outcomes both clinically and service wise for the populations they serve.

Leadership at Neighbourhood Level

Thirdly, we need leadership at primary care level—we need to wrap a range of services around individual patients—therapists, nurses, care staff, general practitioners—making it as easy as possible to navigate the system. We need to keep people as independent as possible for as long as possible—ideally in their own homes if that is what they would want. We need to support people and staff with technology that allows a social worker to talk with a hospital ward clerk, and a practice nurse to talk with a cancer specialist. Above all, we need to adopt the mantra that leadership is as close to the patient as it can be, and only things that cannot be organised individually for a patient should be done at a practice level, or if not there at a neighbourhood level,

ideally with no neighbourhood being bigger than 30,000 to 50,000 population.

A New Deal for the Workforce

Fourthly, we need leadership to tackle the starkly different expectations and motivations of the three generations currently working in the NHS. We need to tackle the emerging workforce crisis in primary care by building up the tripartite staffing structure of care workers, nurses and therapists undertaking extended roles and general medical practitioners. And finally, as the world around us changes ever more quickly through technological change and lifestyle choices, we need an employment offer that remains modern and attractive to the new style NHS worker of the future [6].

Leadership and Promotion of Mental Health Services

Fifthly, we need a new approach to the leadership of mental health services. We need to be moving from quantitative targets to deep meaningful outcome based objectives in this area of care. There is a particular need for leadership talent to be brought to bear on the current unmet mental health needs of young people and to tackle the double epidemic that our children face of childhood obesity and of addressing these mental health problems.

Long Term Planning

Finally, we need leadership that provides a 10 year long term plan for health and care services in this country which is reviewed regularly but is not subject to the short term whims of politicians. The importance of having long term objectives such as 'every person aged 18–24 years in employment, education or training 'within a geographical area should be as important as minimising waiting times for treatment. Of course, any plan needs to be led and delivered by visionary leaders who need some security of tenure in the post to have a fighting chance of success.

Summary

The Independent Commonwealth Fund, based in the US, has ranked the NHS as the top health system performer across 11 countries [7]. The NHS came first in quality, efficiency and cost effectiveness, and came second and third respectively for the timeliness and equity of care. Not a bad record, and one that bodes well for the leadership of the Service tackling the challenges that lie ahead—living longer, changing expectations, workforce shortages, technology and innovation, integrating health and care and the changing socio-economic environment.

But finally I am sure Nye Bevan would say, if he were alive today, none of this matters a jot unless you go back to that simple construct between the giver and receiver of care—and the care and compassion that goes with it, that is the very essence of our NHS and captured so well in the NHS Constitution as follows:

The NHS belongs to the people. It is there to improve our health and well-being, supporting us to keep mentally and physically well, to get better when we are ill and, when we cannot fully recover, to stay as well as we can to the end of our lives. It works at the limits of science-bringing the highest levels of human knowledge and skill to save lives and improve health. It touches our lives at times of basic need, when human care and compassion are what matter most [8].

References

1. 'The New National Health Service' prepared by the Central Office of Information for the Ministry of Health. 1948.
2. Aneuran Bevan; 5 July 1948.
3. Aneuran Bevan. NHS debate 1958 House of Commons 30 July.
4. Times Higher Education. World university rankings. THE; 2015.
5. All-Party Parliamentary Group on Global Health. The UK's contribution to health globally: benefitting the country and the world. APPG-GH; 2015.
6. Facing the facts, shaping the future. A draft health and care workforce strategy for England to 2027. Health Education England.
7. Commonwealth Fund. Mirror on the wall: how the performance of the US healthcare system performs internationally – 2014 update. New York: Commonwealth Fund; 2014.
8. NHS constitution for England. 8 March 2012.

Index